THE corrE

Restoring Beauty
Through Skin Health

AcneC®x -Proofing

An Easy & Proven Way to Prevent Acne Complications & Achieve Clearer Skin Without Injections or Painful Treatments.

A **Scientific, Faith & Wisdom** based Novel Approach!

Acne Scar in Any Face
is One Too many!

Jesse J. Corres, M.D.
Nora M. Corres, RN, BSN

Testimonials and Comments

A novel medical milestone in acne management via paradigm shift in treatment objectives done in an understandable format. instantly translatable to action with visible results.

A handy quick acne reference for ordinary, non medical individuals searching for practical, science based principles and rituals without prescription drugs or invasive procedures.

AcneC®x-Proofing served as a manual for understanding and practicing mitigating principles and processes, which has empowered me a participatory role in creating my own concept of beauty and esthetics.

Thank you Doc. By learning about how acne complications evolve and stopping my unconscious facial bad habits and mannerisms, I see improvements.

AcneC®x-Proofing not only provided practical and doable solutions for my acne but has taught me principles and ideas with profound effect on my life and life style.

As an individual with acne and unfortunately suffering from discoloration, scarring and pigmentations, I feel that reading the PIMPLES AWAY BOOK has given me hope that there is a remedy to prevent and slow down the rapid growth of acne. I already feel my self esteem rising. All is not lost.
The environmental section of PIMPLES AWAY presented a lot of interesting factors and up until this point unbeknown to me. I am never going to chew bubble gum again!

I am one of your patients and I just love your product. I have been using it for 6 months and the change is really amazing. NO MORE PIMPLES!!! I am so happy, thank you.

Testimonials and Comments

Thank you because of you I have hope that I can have a clean, healthy palette without having to put tons of foundation to hide my blemishes. Your book and your products will help people heal not only their scars but also their physical, mental and emotional outlook on life.

My face was always covered with pimples in its various stages of redness, scarring and pigmentations hence I concentrated on pursuing a degree. In spite of having a degree I still could not find a job because of my facial blemishes. Now having used and followed your program for almost 2 years, I not only have a job but also found a husband. Thank you,

I am one of your patients from the Philippines. I just realized that after all these years I never got to thank you so much for introducing me to this amazing treatment program. Dealing with pimples is almost a thing in the past. My relatives and friends have definitely noticed the change, inside and out. (Haha..I sound as if I am testifying from a beauty product ad. Anyhow, I could not thank you enough and ever so much.

AcneC®x-Proofing

Jesse J. Corres, M.D. Nora M. Corres, RN, BSN

Published by

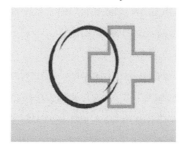

JENOR Publishing LLC
• Chicago •

13-Digit ISBN: 978-1-7378532-0-6

Disclaimer:
This book is designed to provide information about the subject matter covered. The opinions and information expressed in this book are those of the author, not the publisher. Every effort has been made to make this book as complete and as accurate as possible. However, there may be mistakes both typographical and in content. Therefore, this text should be used only as a general guide and not as the ultimate source of information. The author and publisher of this book shall have neither liability nor responsibility to any person or entity with respect to any loss or damage caused or alleged to be caused directly or indirectly by the information contained in this book.

Printed in the United States of America

Dedication

TO THE HOLY TRINITY WHO ALWAYS IS OUR PRIMARY PHYSICIAN AND SURGEON, ON ALL OUR SURGICAL AND NON-SURGICAL ENDEAVORS. TO **HIM** BE THE GLORY FOR MAKING US **HIS** INSTRUMENTS OF LOVE, PEACE AND HEALING. SPECIAL THANKS FOR A JET PROPELLED FINISH OF THIS MANUSCRIPT IN DIGITAL, PRINT AND INTERACTIVE WEBSITE TO COINCIDE WITH OUR 50TH PLUS ONE WEDDING THIS 2021 YEAR, WHICH, IN SPITE OF THE PANDEMIC, WILL ALWAYS LEAVE US WITH INDELIBLE MEMORIES FULL OF GRATITUDE.

TO MY PARENTS FRANCISCO,SR. AND ANACORITA, WHO INCULCATED ON US, SIBLINGS, THE GIFT OF UNCONDITIONAL LOVE. THAT IN ORDER TO ACHIEVE AN ENDURING PEACE OF MIND, ONE HAS TO HAVE PEACE WITH ONESELF, HIS FELLOW MEN AND HIS CREATOR THROUGH LOVE AND SERVICE TO OTHERS. TO BROTHERS DARIO, RAULITO, the late FRANCIS, JR+, SISTERS MERLA, THELMA, LORNA, ROSARIO, NANETTE AND ANNA LEAH.

TO OUR CHILDREN CHRISTINE AND DAVID, JENNIFER AND JASON, JACQUELINE AND LANCE AND OUR GRANDCHILDREN, AVERY CAYLA, CADEN JESSE, ELISE CHRISTINE, RAQUEL, PAYTON, KIERSTIN, REESE LEIGHTON AND CHASE JENSON WHOSE FROLICS AND

ANTICS HAVE GIVEN US A FORE TASTE OF PARADISE AND HEAVEN HERE ON EARTH.

TO OUR PATIENTS FOR THEIR TRUST, LOYALTY AND THE PRIVILEGE OF BEING OF SERVICE TO THEM.

LASTLY, TO MY WONDERFUL, FABULOUS EVER LOVING AND SUPPORTIVE WIFE, **NORA** "NENE" WHO I MAY HAVE NEGLECTED TO SAY "THANK YOU AND I LOVE YOU" AS OFTEN AS I WOULD HAVE LIKE TO. LITERALLY, 'MY PARTNER IN CRIME IN DOING OUR SHARE OF PROVIDING HELP TO THE LEAST OF OUR BRETHREN". SHE IS THE COMPASSIONATE, CARING MOTHER OF MY CHILDREN, DOTING GRANDMA TO OUR GRANDKIDS, ASTUTE BUSINESS PARTNER, EVER-READY SURGICAL NURSE, CRITIC, MODEL AND OFTEN TIMES MY "SPECIMEN-IN-VIVO" FOR MY RESEARCH PROJECTS, MY BEST FRIEND, MY LOVER... MY ALL... MY EVERYTHING... WITHOUT WHOM I WOULD BE JUST A FIGMENT OF WHAT I AM. I LOVE YOU NE, AND THANKS FOR EVERYTHING, ALL THESE YEARS PAST, PRESENT AND THE MANY MORE YEARS TO COME.

TRIPLE "DITTO" AFTER 50 YEARS, NE!!!

Table of Contents

Foreword

Father Adolf Faroni, SDB

A woman without beauty is at a disadvantage; and with beauty has an edge. When we ask girls what they love and desire the most? The common answer will inevitably be: "I dream to be beautiful, I desire beauty and I search for what beauty is. I want to be very beautiful! Not ugly, or a bit beautiful, but beautiful! Beautiful! Beautiful!" And if you ask why? She would answer: "Because God, by using beauty, intended woman to be extremely attractive to men, so that this powerful attraction may result in two loving hearts that unite to love one another and give to the world that heavenly sent being that makes the world so wonderful and joyful: a Baby!

Beauty! Beauty! Beauty! How many hours a girl spends combing her hair, looking at herself in the mirror, searching for that beauty that makes her a kind of angelic creature!

Even if her body might be as beautiful as a heavenly creature, if her face is not beautiful her whole look is spoiled. No man wants an ugly woman, and oh! what a despairing and enduring pain this is to a woman.

Yet, how many are born beautiful and in a short time become ugly by the two enemies of beauty: Acne and Pimples. These deforming enemies of the face can make a beautiful face ugly and repugnant, and this is a daily agony for woman who longs for love!

How many worries, for both men and women, are caused by these ugly intruders. How much discouragement, inferiority complex and sighs are due to to the awareness of a face with beauty destroyed by the two hateful witches: "PIMPLES AND ACNE".

Alas! It would be like heaven if I could uproot the uglifying killers of joy, hopes and of dreams!

However, let us not despair, as a kind voice of science will tell you comforting words: "My dear, do not be depressed, nor lose heart! There is a remedy that can restore the original beauty to your face. Dr. Jesse J. Corres has the transforming secret by which, in a short time, you can do away with "Pimples and Acne" and bring to your face a beautiful smile. In a short time, you can look once more at your face with joy if you read and practice what is recommended in this booklet that all readers love and have at heart to achieve... this much deserved beauty.

Physical beauty is not ever lasting nor eternal. It sadly fades away, yet we are made to be eternally beautiful. When physical beauty has faded due to age, you can still draw out your beauty and be attractive by the beauty of goodness that makes the ugly face of age more beautiful than beauty itself.

Together with the obliteration of the ugly enemies of beauty there is another element that you can add to enhance the beauty of your body and face. Practice virtue, love, compassion and you will add to your physical beauty a spark of the Divine Beauty.

FR. ADOLF FARONI, SDB
Spiritual Adviser and Confessor(RIP)

Foreword

Mila Diloy-Puray, MD, FAACS

As the saying goes, "When you look good, you feel good." And looking good definitely includes having healthy, vibrant skin.

In this book, Dr. Jesse J Corres, a highly esteemed plastic reconstructive and aesthetic surgeon, shares his knowledge, skills and decades of experience and expertise in aesthetics and skin care. He discusses normal skin physiology, the multi factorial causes, pathophysiology of acne, its complications, and how they can be prevented, minimized or corrected.

For the past thirty years Dr. Corres has been immensely successful in treating, correcting, and improving various skin conditions such as pigmentations, wrinkles, solar keratoses, acne, and their complications. These methods are based on the foundation of thorough medical evaluation, intensive patient education, commitment, compliance, and cooperation.

Dr. Jesse Corres offers his highly successful non-invasive corrESthetiques® AcneC®$_{\mathrm{X}}$-Proofing program, a system of topically administered creams and lotions based on skin physiology as a sound, safe and effective way to restore, rejuvenate and maintain healthy skin and vibrant complexion, for your entire life!!!

MILA DILOY-PURAY, MD, FAACS
Board Certified Internist-Hematologist-Sexologist
Mrs. Philippines of Illinois 2007

A Life Time of God-Given Blessings

As the eldest of ten siblings and a humble and public service oriented parentage (public teacher, Anacorita and World War II guerrilla leader, Francisco), we have always been admonished that "if it is worth doing, it's worth doing well even if circumstance might not be at its ideal best." Equipped with an average mind and a steel will determination to succeed, he graduated with honors from Ateneo de Cagayan HS Class1959, now known as Xavier University, Cagayan de Oro City. Various odd jobs such as shoeshine boy, jeepney dispatcher, newspaper and empanada vendor were considered as stepping stones and opportunities for a better future. As a premed student at the same university, his stint as a household helper, masseur, physics and chemistry lab janitor taught him not only the value of money but also the dignity, honor and power of honest labor. He still remembers the late night trips of going home because he can only do these janitorial chores after each physics or chemistry class.

Inspired by a brother, borne with cleft lip and palate and a sister with bilateral cleft lip, Dr. Corres was determined to become a plastic surgeon to find out the cause and treatment of these deformities, so prevalent in the Philippines. After graduating from Cebu Institute of Medicine (formerly CIT College of Medicine), Cebu City, Philippines and passing the Philippine licensing boards that year, he "fly now pay later" to New Jersey, USA as a foreign exchange student. He was recruited by Dr. Abdul H. Islami, Medical Director of Saint

Barnabas Medical Center. This was considered, at that time, as one of the best cleft lip and palate reconstructive centers in the world, and he trained under the tutelage of Dr. Lyndon A. Peer and Dr. John C. Walker for Plastic and Reconstructive Surgery. With added training in Cancer Surgery at Sloane Kettering Memorial Hospital in New York, Dr. Corres moved to Chicago, Illinois where he set up his private practice. He became an attending plastic surgeon in four hospitals, including Mount Sinai Hospital and as an affiliated Assistant Clinical Instructor of surgery, Rush Presbyterian Medical School.

Dr. Corres, an American board certified plastic surgeon, was elected President of the Philippine Medical Association of Chicago in the mid 1980s during which he became the founding President of the International Medical Council of Illinois (IMCI). The IMCI was a coalition of sixteen different ethnic societies of international medical graduates (formerly referred as FMGs) which became the sounding board and lobbying arm against previously xenophobic issues and policies on international medical graduates. These lobbying activities both in Illinois and in the halls of congress in Washington, DC helped paved the way in gaining the respect and parity with its local U. S. counterparts. Other activities include serving as President of the Association of Plastic Surgeons of America; Board Member, Association of Philippine Practicing Physicians of America; American Medical Association, Illinois and Chicago Medical Society; New York Academy of Science; Marquez' Who's Who, International Hair Restoration Society, American Anti-Aging Society, Latin American Association of Cosmetic Surgeons, Philippine Association of Plastic and Reconstructive Surgeons, among other things. He is the recipient of numerous awards and recognitions from medical associations and civic organizations including Rotary, Lions, Zonta Clubs. As a medical volunteer or resource speaker, he journeyed to different parts of the world including Argentina, India, Israel, Japan, Vietnam, Australia, Philippines, and the United States of America.

After doing cosmetic and reconstructive surgery for almost two decades and fully cognizant that surgery or laser alone can not be the answer to facial rejuvenation, he searched the world over and developed JENOR corrESthetiques® skin rejuvenation program. It is a science-based comprehensive, skin restoration program for people wanting to look their best without laser or cosmetic facial surgery. It helps improve skin texture, wrinkles, pigmentation, acne or acne prone skin. Its proper application may prevent warts or sun-related skin blemishes. He authored PIMPLES AWAY, which is becoming a handbook for teens, high school and college students, purposely and mostly written in simple, understandable non "medicalish" format. Its emphasis is on complication prevention (scars, pigmentations, body image changes, etc.) which are almost 100% preventable, as opposed to expecting a cure which is impossible.

Indeed, it has been a lifelong, gratifying journey of labor and love. With pride and humility, assisted by a supportive wife, Dr. Corres was privileged to help his parents educate all his brothers and sisters, including the formerly deformed siblings (now a doctor and a nurse), all successful in their own respective professions. In keeping with his Judeo-Christian principles, he considers it a privilege and a blessing to be able to help level the playing field for the facially deformed specially the marginalized patients. Together with his wife, Nora, their pride and joy is conducting free medical/surgical missions three or four times annually for the past thirty years, where congenitally or traumatically deformed patients are given a second lease on life of having productive and normal lives.

All these things would have been impossible without the help and support of an understanding family. One has to give credit where it is due and that starts with my family, daughters Christine, husband David with children Avery Cayla, Caden Jesse, Elise; Jennifer, husband Jason with children Raquel, Payton, Kierstin, Reese, Chase Jenson; youngest daughter, Jacqueline and husband, Lance. To my wonderful, fabulous and loving wife, Nora, who I may neglect to say

"THANK YOU AND I LOVE YOU" as often as I would like to. She is the compassionate and caring mother of my children, a doting grandma, my ever ready surgical nurse, critic, model and often times my live specimen for my research projects, my best friend, my lover . . . my all . . . MY EVERYTHING.

Together with my wife and family, we give full credit to the ALMIGHTY, the PRIMARY physician/surgeon of all our surgical, medical and socio-civic endeavors. Thank YOU for the privilege of helping our family, our fellowmen, especially the downtrodden, and making us your instruments of HEALING, HOPE, AND PEACE.

Why I am committed to helping others with Acne

O ver a decade has passed since I published the book **ACNE PIMPLES AWAY** in 2007, teaching and showing the reading audience the PRINCIPLES on "how to prevent ACNE COMPLICATIONS rather than CURE acne breakouts." My treatment plan is done without the use of oral medications, painful injections, skin manipulations offered in a spa, beauty salon, or clinic setting. This method is a paradigm shift TO COMPLICATIONS PREVENTION rather than cure.

We have found this particularly helpful for confused teenagers, adults in their twenties, and even adults in their fifties affected by adult onset acne (AOA). The latter is gradually becoming more prevalent due to our current stress-laden lifestyle and environmental pollution. These patients find themselves first using "the usual and customary" anti-acne "quick fixes" and end up confused, frustrated, and disappointed. The widely practiced and oftentimes painful "facial, body cleansing treatments" offered at beauty salons, spas, and doctor's offices, combined with prescribed weeks/months of medications and tedious routines, sadly, result in scarring, pigmentations, and uncontrolled breakouts. Frequently, the patient's impaired appearance leads to anxiety, reduced self-esteem, depression, and sometimes self-mutilation and suicide.

In 2016, the American Acne Society and the American Academy of Dermatology released a guideline on how to treat the various types of acne utilizing prescription and **OTC (over-the-counter)** drugs. Basically, these are chemically and synthetically derived and manufactured medications. On the table below, please notice the three to six drugs under each acne type, an almost automatic and shotgun-like approach by many western educated caregivers.

Courtesy of the American Journal of Dermatology

	Mild	Moderate	Severe
1st Line Treatment	Benzoyl Peroxide (BP) or Topical Retinoid -or- Topical Combination Therapy** BP + Antibiotic or Retinoid + BP or Retinoid + BP + Antibiotic	Topical Combination Therapy** BP + Antibiotic or Retinoid + BP or Retinoid + BP + Antibiotic -or- Oral Antibiotic + Topical Retinoid + BP -or- Oral Antibiotic + Topical Retinoid + BP + Topical Antibiotic	Oral Antibiotic + Topical Combination Therapy** BP + Antibiotic or Retinoid + BP or Retinoid + BP + Antibiotic -or- Oral Isotretinoin
Alternative Treatment	Add Topical Retinoid or BP (if not on already) -or- Consider Alternate Retinoid -or- Consider Topical Dapsone	Consider Alternate Combination Therapy -or- Consider Change in Oral Antibiotic -or- Add Combined Oral Contraceptive or Oral Spironolactone (Females) -or- Consider Oral Isotretinoin	Consider Change in Oral Antibiotic -or- Add Combined Oral Contraceptive or Oral Spironolactone (Females) -or- Consider Oral Isotretinoin

Fig 1. Treatment algorithm for the management of acne vulgaris in adolescents and young adults. The *double asterisks* (**) indicate that the drug may be prescribed as a fixed combination product or as separate component. *BP* Benzoyl peroxide.

I submit that 80 to 85% of EARLY acne cases do not require these drugs for the simple reason that these drugs DO NOT CURE since there has been NO SINGLE IDENTIFIABLE CAUSE of acne that these drugs can readily CURE. Instead, we physicians, should be proactive in educating patients on the prevention of acne complications (NOT cure) and on acne drugs' **supplemental** role. Mindful of the acne guideline authors' disclosures, respected academicians and researchers in their fields, one cannot ignore a semblance of conflict of interest. It is because the researchers/authors and the research medical institutions receive funding or grants from manufacturers of the very drugs that are being researched and investigated. Whatever conclusions and recommendations they make, relevant as they might be, they will always carry a stigma of being tainted and suspect. Their conclusions and recommendations would have carried and commanded more weight had it been peer reviewed by researchers not connected or funded by the manufacturer of these very drugs being studied. Upon review of the entire article, except for two or three sentences, one finds a **glaring lack and deficiency** on strategies PREVENTING ACNE COMPLICATIONS. Very little, if any, mention the PREVENTIVE or MITIGATING ways/efforts of avoiding **acne-induced complications**. These complication signs and symptoms are what make patients seek medical attention. If not properly diagnosed and managed early, such complications can or may lead to devastating results. Such observations have been far too common in both past and present articles, manuscripts, even in standard medical textbooks.

WHY? WHY the lack of emphasis on preventive and mitigating efforts when such measures have been found to be of significant value? This is particularly true in diseases which are multi factorial or its specific cause is unknown or new as in the case of the current COVID-19 pandemic. Deliberate or not, the oversight of effective and helpful strategies on prevention of acne complications, can only trigger misconceptions or sinister speculations unless properly addressed. This might be misconstrued as the medical community's tacit acceptance on because the undercurrent misconception that such advices and counseling have NO significant monetary return and that physicians are in some form of collusion (God forbid) with big pharmaceutical companies.

Identifying the primary cause of any disease and its possible prevention have always been the first and foremost step taken in managing conditions of unknown etiology [the science of causation]. The question is: Are there MITIGATING ways of avoiding these complications which are not only physically deforming but also emotionally and psychologically traumatic? Some might brush off these questions and misconceptions as pure speculations deserving no reply. In my humble opinion, this only aggravates the situation and will not resolve the existing suspicious relationship between physicians and patients. Hopefully, my raising and belaboring these issues on prevention of acne complications will help reconcile the simmering problem of mistrust by offering doable solutions with visible, effective results. I pray that this will encourage and stimulate more discussions and the discovery of more ways of mitigation efforts and rituals. We do need more strategies, although we do have our own, if you allow me to show you how in the subsequent chapters.

But before that, a sincere "Thank You USA" is in order. I may never get this chance to PUBLICLY say THANK YOU for the opportunities and privileges of citizenship without which my dreams would have been in vain. Mindful of the extraordinary responsibilities that US citizenship carries, this provided us HOPE that like minded migrants with determination, excellent work ethics and creative ingenuity can succeed in whatever field we wanted to be or aimed to be. You stood and remained a Bastion of Freedom, particularly, Freedom of Expression of which we are now privileged to use. As much as I love Philippines, my native land, THANK YOU AMERICA, my adoptive country, for being a pathway of what I am today professionally.

As an admirer and lover of things that are beautiful, I am just as resolute in seeking the best and most cost effective solution or solutions for those representing the opposite whether acquired or by birth.

As an aspiring "glorified beautician" looking for the best training ground for restoring facial deformities in the 60s, which country ranks best globally in offering such opportunity? None other than the United States of America! These led me to cross over the Pacific Northwest towards New Jersey and New York to become a certified plastic, reconstructive, cosmetic surgeon, with additional specialized education/training in facial cancer, skin rejuvenation, and integrative medicine in search for doable and science-based beauty solutions in helping restore these afflicted individuals to a state or semblance of normality.

It may seem odd and misguided for a third world native to strive for vanity oriented medical and surgical training. But the birth of my two facially deformed siblings (endemic in the Philippines) started my fascination of beauty. Add to this, the negative social and psychological impact of the absence or maltreatment of tropical skin diseases like leprosy, scabies, and acne on one's self-esteem, observed during medical school, only strengthened my resolve and purpose. Combining medical science with Christian Judaic principles, particularly The Golden Rule, the adoption of my advocacies became easier.

Basically, it is the finding and applying the best solutions for individuals with aesthetic concerns, regardless of cause, to a semblance of normalcy. In addition to taking care of my siblings and other physically challenged patients, I noticed **the scarcity of emphasis on preventive measures** in dealing with acne-related scars and pigmentation, in spite of the prevalence of acne, especially in teens and adult onset acne.

This compeled and obliged me to rewrite ACNE PIMPLES AWAY, now revised as corrESthetiques® AcneC®$_x$-Proofing!

This book is on ACNE COMPLICATIONS PREVENTION, perhaps the only book of its kind that focuses on STEP by STEP prevention strategies, NOT on curing but managing/controlling acne. This is not a book of speculation or imagination. These are evidence-based concepts and techniques starting with a change and shift in treatment direction/paradigm. And that is **from acne cure to acne complications prevention**.

It starts with the patient's awareness and acceptance on the seriousness of one's problem and the willingness to learn how acne complications evolve/develop and is readily managed. Armed with a good understanding of the disease and the meticulous compliance to our suggested acne protocol, one can expect a measurable and visually successful outcome in a matter of days. This is especially enhanced when combined with honest-to-goodness, well reflected, thought-out answers to a goal setting format of WHAT-HOW-WHY?

One may ask, what these W-H-W questions have to do with acne treatment? Honest-to-goodness answers to these questions, when ACTED UPON, have led numerous successful business enterprises, and individuals, to achieve their goals. Why not apply tried and proven concepts in business and lifestyle philosophies to medical cases such as these seemingly innocuous, challenging, and complex **acne vulgaris** cases, especially the stubborn and difficult ones?

I am a board certified reconstructive, cosmetic plastic surgeon with an OBSESSION: To HELP or ALLEVIATE physically, mentally, and spiritually-afflicted individuals. Humbly dubbing myself, a "glorified beautician" servant of Christ, my fascination with "beauty" started with the birth of my two facially deformed siblings in the Philippines.

My Ateneo (Jesuit school), Catholic Christian upbringing and sheer determination helped build and cement the foundation of my goals of finding the best and cost-effective solutions in resolving personal, social, and spiritual challenges faced by these deformed individuals, my siblings included.

Because of their indomitable spirit and firmness of purpose, one sibling became a licensed pediatrician (baby doctor) and the other, a gregarious nurse practitioner. Both earned our family's admiration and the respect of many. Hopefully, their achievements provided a beacon of hope and inspiration to individuals with similar or other deformities.

Physical deformities should NEVER be a hindrance to achieving one's dream, facilitated with providential guidance. Just imagine the consequences, had they not opted to help themselves, but instead wallowed in self-pity, particularly, in a third- world country.

If being blessed to help one's own family is rewarding and fulfilling, how much more for the privilege of uplifting the rest of our brethren? It is an indescribable, heartwarming, sometimes heart-wrenching feeling, especially after aiding people with facial deformities, skin malignancies, and burns. One has to experience it!

It is another reason why I encourage everybody, regardless of profession, to **TRY volunteering** for a medical mission or charitable activity. This act of *loving our neighbor as thyself* **will energize you** as it has promoted others, myself and my wife doing yearly medical missions to the Philippines' poorest of the poor for the past thirty-plus years. As simple as minimizing, hiding, or camouflaging a deforming facial scar evokes an immediate beatific ear-to-ear smile of gratitude that no amount of money can buy.

Although mostly involved in restorative surgery and skin diseases, acne included, these missions confirmed **acne's global incidence**. That such disease does not discriminate age, sex, and economic situation. Mindful of the expensive medications and procedures in treating DEVASTATING acne complications of patients in different parts of the world, PREVENTION OF ACNE COMPLICATIONS BECAME PART OF MY ADVOCACIES.

Truly, a global effort of mitigating acne complications should be advocated in addition to providing affordable medications, especially for the poor.

Actual physical deformity need not be present for anybody to lose self-esteem and self-confidence. A person's psychological or mental issues common in acne patients are just as traumatic and devastating if not immediately and properly addressed. As a plastic and cosmetic surgeon, I have seen and treated the physical facial ravages of acne that even in the best of methods, fail to meet the expectations of both patients and treating physicians. Their unpredictable results, expenses incurred from frequent office visits/procedures and permanent loss of time, compelled me to raise public awareness to the great importance of ACNE COMPLICATIONS PREVENTION methods.

It is NOT ABOUT PREVENTING ACNE FROM HAPPENING, but the PREVENTION OF PERMANENT ACNE COMPLICATIONS. I firmly believe "A SINGLE SCAR due to acne in anybody's face, IS ONE TOO MANY!"

As a Christian physician, I consider it a privilege and a blessing to be able to combine medical science and faith-based strategies to best help alleviate a patient's health and beauty concerns.

Dr. Albert Einstein, perhaps, 20th century's greatest scientist, an atheist himself, once declared that science without religion is lame. But religion without science is blind.

Armed with a healthy dose of common sense and science-based precepts under the Great Healer's guidance we have, with confidence, helped resolve such challenges.

Did you know that the Holy Bible mentions numerous healing verses. The word "Heal" appears 40 times and the word "Healed" 79 times! Why is it that we ONLY seek God's help in the midst of difficulties and often times, when things seem totally hopeless? Why not seek guidance or help BEFORE the onset of a project/problem?

A heavy load always feels lighter when carried with SOMEONE, especially if that someone cares for you. Did you know that patients CONSENSUALLY being prayed over by their physicians have been shown to recover faster as compared to those not being prayed over?

By analogy, business hedge fund managers are PAID to manage and astutely plan preventive measures to lessen the impact of an unforeseen portfolio decline or debacle. Who better or best can we call on health issues/crisis but the Best Healer of all times, JESUS!

All we have to do is "ASK and YOU SHALL RECEIVE. SEEK AND YOU SHALL FIND."

Traditional therapy entails making a diagnosis based on history and symptoms, followed by treatment usually with the use of chemicals or prescription drugs.

With the advent and popularity of wellness programs, more and more individuals are into a proactive mode of "HOW TO PREVENT" disease and its complications. Unfortunately, not much has been written on the precluding and mitigating aspects of acne complications. In case of acne, where there is NO cure, emphasis should focus on methods, strategies, and measures on how to prevent acne complications.

This book therefore teaches methods and ways of how to prevent/ avoid permanent acne complications as opposed to "CURING" of the acne disease, where there is NONE.

Acne: The Number One Skin Disease

Doctors call it the **NUMBER #1** skin disease affecting teenagers all over the world as **8 out of 10 teenagers** are afflicted with it. In fact **85%-95% of all adults, worldwide**, have suffered some form of acne sometime in their life. Scientifically termed as **acne vulgaris**, layman label it as: pimple, acne, **zit**, breakout, **teenager's plague** or a curse. Acne used to be "just part of the growing up phenomenon" but has now evolved into a perplexing, embarrassing, and increasingly common, frustrating skin condition occurring even in adults! The complications of improperly treated or untreated acne are devastating, resulting in scarring that may become permanently deforming, both physically and emotionally. **Acne sufferers** have been shown to exhibit **problems** of **low self-esteem, low self-confidence, social withdrawal, misconceived body image, depression** and, in some cases, self-mutilation and suicide. All of us recognize what acne is because we all suffered its effect sometime in our life. This can vary from a single lesion to widespread appearance of **papulopustular cystic eruptions** in the face, neck, chest and back. These breakouts are statistically more common in females than in males, with eruptions being worst a week before or during their menstrual period, thus confirming its **hormonal influence**. Other **factors** appearing **to have considerable influence on the incidence of acne are:** *genetics or hereditary predisposition, *diet, *stress, *drugs and *improperly applied topical acne products**. Because of these numerous influential factors it would be a mistake for any physician and, more so, other non medical, self-proclaimed skin health providers (with their "revolutionary concoctions") to claim a treatment that will totally "cure" acne as there is NONE. On the other hand, with early diagnosis and treatment, physicians can certainly avoid and minimize, the complications of acne which include **scarring, pigmentations, misconceptions of body image, depression** and **low self-esteem**. These can only be achieved by discarding the old restrictive role of, "Me, doctor and healer; You, patient ONLY" relationship. It is this "God Complex" attitude of doctors that may oftentimes hinder the success of acne management. A **compassionate, interactive doctor-patient partnership** must be established to achieve the best skin-health regimen of one's acne, especially those affecting the face. It is therefore imperative that **empathetic physicians** take time in educating and informing patients **what patients must DO** and **NOT DO**. They should not just prescribe anti-acne medications after a brief and cursory physical examination. Successful treatment of acne patients can only be achieved when there is mutual trust, understanding and cooperation between the doctor and patient.

What better time and chance of controlling acne than now because of recent medical advances and innovations. These include a better understanding of acne's pathophysiology (how acne behaves and develops), its diagnosis and latest therapeutic advances. Yet, why are so many innocuous skin blemishes, acne scars, pits and pigmentations still an everyday occurrence among today's teenagers and even in adults? I would like to share some insights, observations and treatment options that are not "break through" but a **"break with" current** and **traditional acne treatment** that the **corrESthetiques®** AcneC®$_X$-Proofing have used with great success for more than 30 years. It is without injections or any of those invasive or manipulative procedures commonly done in a beauty salons or even in doctor's offices. Let me caution the lay public that it is challenging enough for doctors to treat and control acne, how much more for the layman or ordinary non medical person. Patients, who are not confident enough or sure of what they have, should never put upon themselves the burden of self-medication as it is froth with high incidence of failure. They should get a medical consultation when in doubt and especially when dealing with facial acne. An initial honest-to-goodness consultation with an **empathetic and compassionate physician "on the know"** will go a long way. Better still, if that physician or care giver actively preaches and practices the **NEW** treatment paradigm shift principles of: Acne Complications Prevention. In short, the corrESthetiques® AcneC®$_x$-Proofing protocol.

What is corrESthetiques® AcneC®x-Proofing?

J ust as there is water-proofing, rust-proofing and even age-proofing, I humbly suggest that a comprehensive, science and evidence-based **paradigm shift** [radical change in one's way of thinking] **in acne treatment** be initiated and that it be called corrESthetiques® AcneC®x-Proofing. In medical parlance, Rx symbolizes treatment/therapy; Px physical examination; Dx diagnosis and for simplicity sake, I will use AcneCx® as a shortened symbol of acne complication.

Our acne management focuses on the **prevention** of acne complications as opposed to that of curing acne. How can a physician or caregiver assure an acne patient a "cure" when major **contributory factors** like, *genetics, *erratic hormonal changes and the very challenging *stress factor have NO known specific therapy? Let's contrast this with **controlling** a few **acne complications** such as: **infection, *scarring, *pigmentations, *psychological issues like misconceived body image** and **depression** that can certainly be minimized if not totally avoided. In spite of the recent innovations and advancement in acne management, complications galore persist. This can perhaps be attributed to the still **pervasive** but WRONG acne treatment objective, which is "**acne cure instead of acne complications prevention**". In our office therefore, we have developed a step by step procedure, the main purpose of which is the prevention of the complications to occur or worst, for them to become permanent. Although "cured acne cases" have been sporadically reported, NO single drug has claimed to do such feat. However, a combination of pharmaceuticals have been recommended which sometimes, sadly, lead to disastrous outcomes, especially when used by the uneducated. The reason for this failure is obviously the MULTIFACTORIAL influences on acne such as, genetics, hormonal changes, stress and even ill advised local facial rituals. It is simply futile to aim for cure because there is NONE, "NADA", "NYET"! It is just the big pharmaceuticals and medical equipment company's gain, with their ever unending expensive acne medications and instrumentations. Compared to the current corrESthetiques® AcneC®$_X$-Proofing treatment **approach that focuses on acne complications prevention**, the objectives are definitely doable and achievable. This is especially true with early and proper education and practicing science based preventative and mitigating efforts initially. These may or may not require judicious use the over the counter pharmaceuticals and less invasive procedures as supplements.

It has been proven that properly informed patients, undergoing a surgical or simple medical treatment, have a better chance of a successful outcome, compared to the uninformed. For this reason, educating and informing the patient is usually done on the first consultation wherein the **patient and the doctor** have a chance of exchanging ideas and establishing information on the following questions: What is the duration and nature of the acne problem? What is the planned approach? What are the potential risks and complications? What are the treatment options-both preventive and therapeutic? What are the cost(s) involved? All these practical questions might be all very important but one has to really involve the patient himself/herself. Very often when patients are asked, "why are you in my office?" The retort is, "I don't know. My Mom or grandma brought me here!" These types of patients are surely bound to fail unless patients ACCEPT or are AWARE THAT THEY HAVE AN ACNE PROBLEM. Empathetic doctors and care givers should help identify such issues with mirrors and photographs. Only then, do we encourage them to commit to a simple and measurable goal setting format in addition to the corrESthetiques® AcneC®x-Proofing program. It has been said, "where there is no vision, people perish". Hence, we encourage a participative role on all our patients. This is done by, almost fanatically, keeping them tuned in to an imaginary radio station, **WHW - FM**. The **WHAT-HOW-WHY** question station. Well reflected and honest-to-goodness answers to these **WHW** questions have been the core and essence of almost all successful businesses and individuals, personally experienced by many of our compliant patients.

To illustrate how to use the **WHW**, on a personal note, I am the oldest of 10 siblings from a third world country. Before I reached high school, I was exposed to the shocking and difficult parental and brotherly rigors of helping raise a brother born with a complete cleft lip and palate. This is a condition where the lip muscles and the bony roof of the mouth have failed to fuse or merge with the opposite side, thus leaving a gap or a cleft and its accompanying feeding and speaking difficulties. This was followed by a sister born with bilateral cleft lip after a few years. Both events, after a period of compassionate adjustments, stirred up my first thought of becoming a doctor, which became my **W** or WHAT is my OBJECTIVE/GOAL in life. What started as a shocking experience, combined with my inquisitive mind of why these facial deformities happen, reinforced my initial interest of helping the facially deformed. The ultimate goal of finding ways to prevent, repair, reconstruct and rehabilitate to normalcy facial deformities was so compelling that at such a young age I decided: I HAVE TO BE A PLASTIC SURGEON. The following question I posed: "how do you plan to achieve such a goal on an average (IQ) mind, and (being eldest of 10 siblings) on LIMITED educational funds coming from your parent's combined public school teacher and civil engineer salaries?" And as the saying goes, "if there is a will, there is a way" anchored on the firm and supreme belief of the Almighty's guidance and help.

The **H** or HOW are the METHODS/STRATEGIES employed to achieve TANGIBLE and MEASURABLE RESULTS that can instantly judge failure or success. A medical degree requires: grades to be above average in high school and premed, passing the MCAT exams before admittance to a local 5-year medical school. Results of the various requisite exams, serve as measurable parameters for an individual's chance of achieving his/her goal of becoming a future plastic surgeon. This is a medical specialty that deals with restoring congenital, traumatic and acquired defects of the body to a physical semblance of normality and function. It requires additional years of training, usually, from another country, which was the United States of America, after graduating from the local medical school. The financial burden—bank loans, "fly now pay later plane fare schemes", the loneliness from family separation, the hurdle of passing another set of required examinations for specialty eligibility, in another advanced foreign country, together with cultural adjustments to it, make the challenge even more formidable. With proper attitude, perseverance and determination, the effort becomes worthwhile and filled with great satisfaction. It even becomes sweeter and more fulfilling when such WHW blue print are previously put in writing and witnessed by family or anybody to monitor and verify. With God's grace, I was able to finish my Plastic surgery training at Saint Barnabas Medical Center, Livingston, New Jersey under the tutelage of the legendary Dr. Lyndon A. Peer and his group. Their work on facial deformities and tissue transplantation were pioneering and were achieved while Dr. L. Peer was the editor-in-chief for the national Journal of the American Society of Plastic and Reconstructive Surgeons, a position which he held until his retirement.

The **W** or WHY is perhaps the most important item to address, as this becomes the individual's COMPELLING and INSPIRING reason of "WHY you are AIMING for such a goal?" Such intention usually goes beyond financial/monetary goals. Goals based on amassing fortune have been found by many to have no end to such quests, some of them ending in dismal failure. Instead, I set a goal more noble and with a higher level of purpose. I made obtaining knowledge and sharing the "technical know-how" of managing and repairing facial and other body deformities my goals. These have allowed me the privilege of helping not only my siblings, but other patients afflicted with similar deformities in my country, a more inspiring and fulfilling purpose, indeed. Together with my ever supportive wife, Nora, who is also a surgical nurse, we are humbled, blessed and privileged to do all these things, which has become a yearly and still ongoing labor of love for 35+ years (and more, God willing) of joining medical missions with various local and international groups as our share of "helping the least of our brethren". All of us 10 siblings attained our individual chosen professions, THANKS, most especially, to the ever loving Almighty God, and my parents who will always be my original idols. My two facially deformed siblings became my added idols because of what they attained for themselves, one becoming a successful pediatrician (baby doctor) and the other a nurse practitioner each with successful families of their own. They would have not succeeded without a clear and goal oriented WHW plan of their own.

In our incessant dreams to improve ourselves and become successful, most sages often advise to study and reflect on the history and lives of successful people and enterprises. Individuals like WBA champion Manny Pacquiao, literally an under educated street child, the ONLY 8-title-holder in 8 different world boxing divisions, Steve Jobs of Apple, The Wright Brothers (Orville and Wilbur), inventor of the motor driven airplane and father of Aviation. Corporations like Amazon, Google, Facebook and Alibaba are just examples to name a few. All of them used or tuned in to the WHW-FM goal setting station in various forms or another in order to succeed. The principles remain the same for the BIG 3 WHW QUESTIONS. One has to answer the **WHAT**: the (objectives) of one's goals are clear and well defined; the **HOW**: (methods/strategies) to execute [to carry out fully] your plan [a detailed formulation of a program of action] to achieve your objectives. Metrics or measurable ways **must** be used to monitor one's success or failure. Lastly, the **WHY**: the (reason) SHOULD be a compelling, inspiring vision that goes beyond the usual money or financial motivation. When written, and clearly inculcated in one's mind, failure becomes remote. This is especially true and more meaningful when your WHW are made in the presence of friends/family and WITNESSED by a chosen few.

Any endeavor will be subject for failure unless basic WHW principles are met, be it in medical or non medical issues. One should NEVER be afraid of failure so long as he/she realizes that most of these failures, when duly identified and corrected, are essential stepping stones towards eventual success. And this holds true with our approach in dealing with acne. Very often, treatment failure happens because of making wrong objectives, just like "a dog barking up at the wrong tree" or an individual, steering a rudderless boat. I submit that current acne treatment plans, which aims for cure, when there is NONE, is based on the WRONG premise/objective. The high and common incidence of devastating complications, despite scientific advances and innovations, obligate us to change our treatment paradigm from **acne cure** to acne **complication prevention**. Let us focus more on measurable strategies that are almost 100% achievable in precluding acne complications. Supplement these with early basic skin health education and the practice of Good Morals and Conduct and we have a win-win situation. Let's Think PREVENTION via EDUCATION!

You as a patient, are paying that doctor for his time and expertise. It is your legal right to be as fully informed about your medical problem regardless of time. Treatment should not be just a cursory exam followed by a written prescription of acne medications to be taken for a few weeks. One should not be shy in asking your doctor pertinent questions regarding your acne issues. Should there be any doubt with your current doctor's ability to handle such questions, then, you should not hesitate to seek a SECOND OPINION from another medical practitioner.

Treating acne for that matter should be no different. The corrESthetiques® AcneC®$_x$-Proofing program or protocol begins with a detailed history and physical examination. This is followed with a quick overview about acne, its causes, evolution and suggested treatment and the time frame involved for a visual result. Mandatory "before treatment" photos of the patient from the patient's smart phone or office camera are then taken.

Let me begin by **defining acne**, which is a combination of acute and chronic inflammation of the **pilose**[1] [*hairy*] -**sebaceous**[2] glands of various degrees.

SKIN ANATOMY

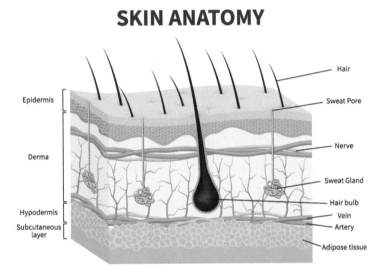

Ideally, our **sebaceous**[1] [*secreting sebum or other fatty material*] glands, which are located in the dermis[2] [*(the sensitive vascular inner layer of) the skin*], next to the hair follicle[3] [*a small anatomical cavity or deep narrow depression*], secrete the right amount of oil or sebum. This oil is emptied into a canal-like structure which is called the hair **follicle canal**, and this canal goes out to the outer skin, via the skin pore, to lubricate and moisturize the skin and make the hair shiny. Everyday there is a continuous shedding or peeling-off of the lining of the **follicular canal**, which is directly adjacent to[4] the outer skin layer.

Under normal circumstances, the oil or sebum is mixed with the daily shed dead cells within the **follicular canal** and channeled to the outer skin without difficulty. In unhealthy skin such as with acne, there is an excessive amount of oil production and excessive shedding or peeling-off of dead cells of both the lining of the **follicular canal** and outer skin, which when mixed together create a plug. This plug, as it travels towards the outer skin, can clog the skin pore. This sometimes becomes the early stage of the development of an acne comedy.

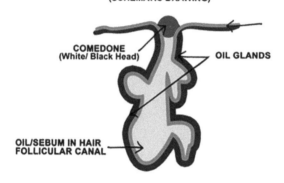

EVOLUTION OF ACNE COMEDO
(SCHEMATIC DRAWING)

COMEDONE
(White/ Black Head)

OIL GLANDS

OIL/SEBUM IN HAIR
FOLLICULAR CANAL

Notice the **top layer** or **epithelium** [*a usually thin layer of cells that lines a cavity*] of the skin (green color) that is continuously connected to the lining of the **follicular canal**. It is this constant peeling off of this layer combined with the excess oil production that contributes to the frequent clogging of the skin pores, resulting in the formation of **comedo**. It is called a **whitehead** or **closed comedo** when the dead cells and sebum inside the **follicular canal** forms a plug and is blocked by the skin pore so that it cannot expose the plug to the air. It is called a **blackhead** or **open comedo** when the plug of dead cells and sebum has distended[1] the skin pore, exposing the plug to the air changing the colour of the contents into a dark colour which is not dirt but a melanin[2] [*a dark brown or black animal and plant pigment (eg of skin or hair)*] pigmentary[3] oxidation[4] reaction. Within the **follicular canal** and the outer skin are normal **bacterial inhabitants**[5], like **propionibacterium acnes (p.acnes)**, which are harmless when the skin integrity[6] is intact (not damaged). If the

follicular canal wall breaks from the gradual distension[7] of its contents, then inflammation[8] sets in due to the invasion of **p.acnes** and other **bacteria**. As **bacterial invasion** sets in together with the foreign body reaction against the plug of dead cells and sebum or oil, varying degrees of inflammation resulting in painful papules[9] [*pimples*], pustules[10] [*a pimple containing pus*] and cysts[11] develop. These cystic, nodular[12] inflammatory[13] lesions[14] can sometimes lead to permanent pigmentations and scarring which in the long run can lead to a **psychological overlay**[15] such as depression or **suicide** if not properly managed.

In short, **acne breakouts involve a combination of multiple factors** and not just one single factor. They include: 1) the abnormal keratinization of the skin and **follicular canal**, 2) the hyperactivity of the sebaceous glands, 3) the colonization of the **propionibacterium acnes (p.acnes)** leading to the release of inflammatory mediators into the skin, ie sebaceous lipids and metalloproteinases (MMPs). A total treatment or cure of acne has NOT yet been established, because no single direct cause and effect relationship factor has been identified. Rather, there are multitude of influences1, both inherent2 and external3 that cause acne. This is why for any clinical doctor or beauty salon advertisement, whether in TV, radio or in print, claiming to possess a complete, curative acne treatment is not only a misleading statement but utterly false!

In the past several years, the pathogenesis of acne have not only changed the name of **Propionibacterium acnes (p.acnes)** to **Cutibacterium** acnes as the causative agent but also debate continues as to whether inflammation/infection occur before or after **comedo** formation. These changes however will have little to NO bearing in our approach to acne management, which is concentrated on complications prevention.

Acne cure has to be differentiated from acne control, which is not only feasible but also very much achievable. It is towards this latter goal that our acne treatment program has been based on for over 30 years with good to excellent results. I believe it is safe to state that although **THERE IS NO TOTAL CURE FOR ACNE, the major COMPLICATIONS OF ACNE CAN CERTAINLY BE PREVENTED**. Fifty to 80% of these cases might not require rigid medical supervision. In fact, the early or mild forms of acne (which comprise the majority of these cases) can be controlled with a properly oriented goal and determined effort of self-education on basic skin care, and judicious use of **over-the-counter** (OTC) anti-acne products. The question seems to be, if management is seemingly that simple then *"why are acne scarred patients with their accompanying physical, mental suffering and anguish still very common in today's society?"* It is because acne is so deceptively harmless when it starts, that individuals take them for granted! Acne is largely ignored, or at best haphazardly1 discussed as just part of adolescence and "part of the growing-up phenomenon". Unfortunately by the time individuals take notice of their acne, severe skin damage has already set in, resulting in ugly **facial pigmentations, scarring, low self-esteem** and **body image problems**. Moreover, since we live in a society that puts a high premium on appearance especially a "youthful and blemish free appearance", putting on one's best face forward becomes more urgent. We have placed high values on facial appearance and self-confidence, attributes that are severely affected and devastating by mismanaged or untreated acne. I believe **BASIC FACIAL SKIN CARE AND GROOMING SHOULD BE PART OF THE INTERMEDIATE GRADE OR HIGH SCHOOL CURRICULUM** to save these individuals from the agonizing and sometimes dehumanizing effects of acne complications.

A proactive, massive public awareness, through education and mentoring with emphasis on PREVENTION can minimize, if not eliminate, these acne complications. What better time to start this campaign than in their intermediate junior and high schooling while still in possession of flawless and healthy skin. If I, as a physician or teacher, can prevent one child from developing the stigma or scourge of acne/pimple complications, then I would have considered writing this treatise a worthwhile effort. It is also for this very reason that our main target audience are the mild and moderate acne sufferers, educating them on preventative measures before these complications become permanent.

Let me begin by sharing with you how we manage acne patients that come to our office. At the outset, I want to categorically1 state that in no instance do I claim this as a "sure how to" medical guide especially for non-physicians, but rather to be used as acne BASIC reference or an alternative approach to some currently available treatments. Patients should NOT construe the information rendered herein as reasons to avoid physician-prescribed medications and laboratory tests. Hopefully, this presentation will help enlighten and empower the affected public sector to **practice** the **PRINCIPLE OF CHOICE**. You have the power to select your physician and his services, as much as you have the power to choose the type of face you want: will it be acne-scarred or not by following corrESthetiques® AcneC®x-Proofing algorithm?

Would you want to have an acne-studded and scar-disfigured face shown in Figure A. and Figure B. or, would you like to try a science based and proven way of avoiding such scars and pigmentations? Practicing the principle of your right to choose, I encourage you to take part in a proactive treatment program that helps eliminate these complications significantly, if not totally.

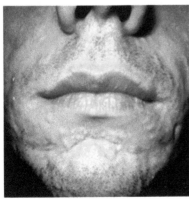

Figure A   **Figure B**

Are there ways of avoiding or preventing these above shown scars as well as their accompanying pigmentations? Once developed, can these scars and pigmentations be corrected or treated? The answer to these questions is a qualified "**YES**" regardless of age.

Management begins by the patient's **acceptance** or **awareness** that she or he has an acne problem. This is followed by identifying contributing factors1 of acne, especially, those that are damaging but controllable. A review of those uncontrollable factors need to be discussed.

Uncontrollable Factors (influences) of Acne

GENETICS

Certainly, a genetically acne prone individual does not have any choice of being born to a couple with a genetic acne predisposition. There is not much anyone can do about the abnormally excessive shedding of dead cells, which includes the lining of the **follicular canal** and the outer skin. The excessive sebum/oil production of the sebaceous glands, when combined with the excessive shedding of dead cells, and the lining of the **follicular canal** and outer skin; along with the increase[1] of resident anaerobic[2] [an organism (eg a bacterium) that lives only in the absence of oxygen] **bacteria**, forms a plug composed of dead cells and sebum that can trigger the beginning of an acne eruption.

Abnormally excessive shedding of dead cells (of both the lining of **follicular canal** and outer skin) + excessive sebum/oil production + multiplication of **propionibacterium acne (p.acnes)** and anaerobic bacteria = **formation of acne.**

TYPES OF ACNE PIMPLES

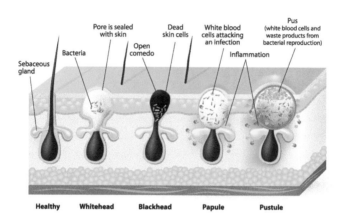

Although genetic engineering is now feasible, such high-tech or advance science methodology is not yet applicable in acne management. We do not have any control over these genetic influences at this point. However, we should not despair since genetics is just one of the contributing acne factors. Instead of blaming parents for one's unfortunate lot or situation, identifying these controllable factors contributing to acne becomes of paramount importance. Among these **multi-factors (ie influences contributing to** a result or **incidence) of acne** are the following: *medications, *hormones, *diet, *environmental factors, and *bad, repetitive, self-destructive, clinic or salon induced facial manipulations and treatments.

Alterable and Modifiable Factors (influences) of Acne

I. DIET

II. BAD REPETITIVE FACIAL HABITS AND SKIN PRACTICES

III. ENVIRONMENTAL FACTORS

IV. HORMONAL OR ENDOCRINE DISORDERS

V. MEDICATIONS : DIFFERENT APPROACHES IN THE TREATMENT OF ACNE

I.   DIETARY CONCERNS

Does diet have anything to do with the development of acne? Reports of a particular native or tribe in **Paraguay** and **New Guinea** whose diets involve a **low glycemic index** or low carbohydrate intake, were found to have very **low non incidence of acne**. These reports have not been fully validated. Although there are certain individuals with food sensitivities that trigger the appearance of acne eruptions, an attempt to identify these particular food culprit(s)[1] would be the best thing to do. If one can discover a cause and effect relationship between a particular food and the appearance of acne, then it is logical and appropriate for the individual to avoid those particular foods or drinks. These may include common items as caffeine, chocolate, nuts, spicy food and even dairy products. However, to have a blanket statement[2] that "all individuals should avoid eating the above mentioned food stimulants" for fear of acne eruption is definitely uncalled for if they have not found a definitive cause and effect relationship. Besides, to embark on an **elimination diet** may actually cause an **increase of acne eruptions because of stress due to the release of cortisol** and **adrenaline**[3]. This is why restrictive and fad diets are usually not advisable because of the possibility of aggravating acne. **Seaweeds, some fish** (perch, cod, sea bass), **shellfish**; **vegetables** such as spinach, artichoke, kale, onions, mushrooms, lettuce, green peppers; **fruits** (pineapple); **some vitamins and minerals and processed food** —because of its high iodine content— have been associated with acne development or its exacerbation[1]. **Brominated**[2] soft drinks have similar effect.

Treatment therefore includes identifying the offending food/drink and their avoidance. Even milk, which has shown to increase the risk of acne break outs have to be minimized or stopped. For stubborn type of acne, food(s) that have high **glycemic** index (high in **sugar** content) may have to be avoided. This food leads to **hyperinsulinemia** leading to the production of the comedogenic IGF-1 [insulin-like Growth Factor-1 Hormone]. Medical studies have reported improvement of inflammatory lesions with the use of the trace mineral, **zinc**. Supplementary or replacement zinc therapy 15 mg per day prevents the conversion of **testosterone** to **dihydrotestosterone** (**DHT**), a sebum-stimulating hormone, a major cause of acne development.

II.   BAD REPETITIVE FACIAL HABITS AND RITUALS

BAD REPETITIVE FACIAL HABITS AND SKIN PRACTICES, SHOULD ALL BE BANNED AND STOPPED IF POSSIBLE! THESE CAN LEAD INTO NEEDLESS PHYSICAL AND EMOTIONAL MISERIES.

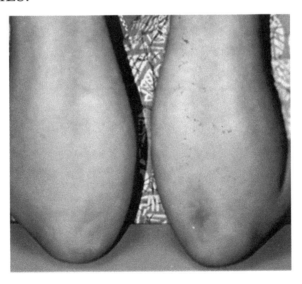

Pigmentation of the left elbow due to repeated scratching

Let us begin with myths and half-truths about how one washes one's face. Individuals should **not wash their face more than twice a day**. Doing so will just **decrease the natural body defenses** of the skin thereby aggravating the individual's problematic skin condition.

Facial scrubbing or rubbing with the use of the hand or any coarse or **abrasive materials** such as salt scrubs, **granules**, grains, **loofahs**, pumice or towels will not make your skin any smoother or cleaner. In fact, it might cause more harm than help, especially on acne prone skin. These patients have already hyperactive oil/sebaceous glands, which when **massaged** or manipulated will just cause enlargement or hypertrophy[1]of these glands. Basic medical physiology dictates that when you stimulate a gland or muscle this will make the gland bigger and the muscle bulkier. This is like going to the gym or health club, that when you exercise your muscles they get bigger and bulkier. Stop exercising for a few days and they get smaller. This is another basic and proven observation in medical science: "If you don't use it or stimulate it, you lose it". This is called the "**Principle of atrophy or dis-use**".

What does this principle have to do with acne management? Because of the known hyperactivity of the **pilo-sebaceous** glands, **avoiding** or minimizing skin stimuli thru **vigorous washing**, **rubbing or massaging** to create suds and bubbles, has lead our observation of a much more smoother, radiant and clearer skin. This can be attributed to the "**principle of atrophy or dis-use**" or "if you don't use it, you lose it". We, therefore, recommend the gentle application of our creams and lotions —enough pressure to spread them not massage them in. Acne and acne prone patients should use **synthetic detergent**-cleansers that work on enzymatic or foaming action with the skin. By using foam and enzymatic detergent, it loosens dirt, oil, and dead cells, without vigorous rubbing or scrubbing after a very short and gentle application on the skin. This is followed by splash rinsing or submerging the face in a basinful of lukewarm or tepid water. A foaming gel will also serve the same purpose so long as the foam suds or bubbles are not generated by vigorous scrubbing or rubbing. The objective being, to eliminate or minimize the stimulation of the already hyperactive **pilo-sebaceous** glands.

For those unable to find high-tech **synthetic detergent**, any cleanser or liquid soap will suffice, keeping in mind the importance of handling or touching the skin gently and gingerly. **Caution** ought to be used on **bar soaps**, designer or not. They have **NO place** in acne skin care regimen because the ingredient used to convert that liquid soap to its solid form has been reported as acnegenic or comedogenic (clogging of skin pore).

THE ROLE OF FACIAL MASSAGE, COMEDO EXTRACTION (WHITEHEAD OR BLACKHEAD REMOVAL), and MASK USE ON ACNE PRONE PATIENTS

After giving patients basic information of how acne develops and behaves, we DO NOT encourage the use of the above services especially when done aggressively and vigorously. **Facial massage** may physiologically enhance the already hyperfunctioning **sebaceous/oil** gland of an acne/acne prone skin thereby increasing its oil production! It is important to inform patients that **whitehead and blackheads are not dirt and will comeback every 2 to 3 weeks after extraction** as part of a patient's skin abnormality. Except for a semblance of temporary facial cleanliness, removing and extracting can actually cause more problems if not done professionally under supervision. First, there is that REALISTIC DANGER (although remote) of getting AIDS and other infections from indiscriminate or improper use of **contaminated needles and extractors**. While we are on the topic of realistic danger medical students are taught, early on in their medical education, about an area in the face called the **"dangerous triangle of the face"**. This is an area in the central part of the face occupied by the nose and its immediate skin surroundings. The very close proximity to the **brain** especially in relation to its local circulation and blood supply, could cause the spread of local infection. Any form of pimple, acute or chronic, has the potential of spreading to the **brain** that may lead to its infection and its membranes. How can this be prevented? Inflammation or infection in this area should be handled with extreme care and caution, medical supervision when in doubt. As for prevention of AIDS, insist on the use of **sterile disposable needles** and gloves.

Even in the best of hands, when **extracting comedoe**[1], accidental pricking/puncture of the skin occurs. Bleeding—gross or microscopic—can lead to pigmentation, infection followed by scarring, in other words, a cascade of reactions that are very **common sequelae**[2] of these seemingly innocuous procedures. Unless done repeatedly, the facial skin is very forgiving when it comes to healing, thus leaving neither permanent scarring or pigmentation. However, if the skin incursions, scratches, trauma, etc. are **repetitive**, as in **"acne self-picking or self-squeezing"**, which most of acne patients habitually do, **then permanent disfiguring** scars and pigmentation occur. It is interesting to note that although acne scars are small, shallow, and pitted, it is the associated pigmentations that make them very noticeable. An important consideration in improving the acne scar pigmentation should not only be directed on prevention, on the harmful effects of sun exposure through judicious use of sun protectors, on sun protection, but also neutralizing the pigmentary effects of hemoglobin [the red oxygen-carrying pigment in the red blood corpuscles] breakdown (**hemosiderin**)[3]. If a patient picks his or her acne once, even if associated with bleeding, no permanent pigmentation arises because their local skin circulation can absorb the by-products of inflammation and hemoglobin breakdown. However, if the picking and **squeezing habits** are repetitive, these traumatic pigmentations accumulate and get darker, deeper and harder to control. (I will discuss this further in the treatment section at a later chapter). AVOIDANCE ON THESE PROCEDURES OBVIOUSLY IS THE BEST SOLUTION to prevent these potential acne complications. An alternative to removing whitehead and blackheads will be the use of **retinoid**[4], exfoliants, topically applied **adhesive strips,** with caution.

These strips are particularly useful for teenagers but its use has to be used with caution when applying to the older age group because of the skin's fragility. **Bimonthly or monthly facial mask** applications may also be of benefit particularly the **clay cleansing type** which contain **sulphur, bentonite, aluminum,** etc. which are all **absorbents**. This cleansing mask has to be **differentiated** from the **moisturizing type** which contain **polymers of polyester** which might **be comedogenic**.

Because this requires a 20 or 30 minutes application time, this might be the best time to employ some **meditation or visualization** with positive affirmations. Since these do not include massage manipulations that invade the skin's integrity, complications are virtually absent if not minimized.

Even if we strongly advise our patients to refrain from touching/ stroking their face, particularly when acne eruption is present, such habit is almost impossible to comply. Acne patients have developed that **sense of euphoria** or well being when they get to see a blackhead come out or a white, cheesy material come out from a "**good squeeze of the nose**". For those who have the **urge to squeeze**, especially in the presence of inflammation, although we absolutely discourage it, permit me to give some patient **guidelines on how to do it properly**.

First, be sure to wash your hands properly. Second, **wash your face GENTLY** to soften the skin. Third, employing the soft pads of two fingers (avoiding the nail tip) apply gentle pressure (i.e. with the minimum amount of pressure) just beyond the affected site - for a few seconds; if the plug comes out easily and freely then you can repeat the same maneuver to the other affected areas. If it takes a heavier **squeeze of more than 5 to 10 seconds, and requires squeezing more than twice, with still no plug coming out, then STOP because it will not come out with more finger pressure**. In fact it will just trigger inflammation and possibly begin new pimple formations along with consequences. NOTE: If the area of concern now appears reddened and inflamed then you have applied to much pressure and you should STOP immediately! This self-squeezing should not be done more often than every 14 days.

The **early acne** spots just beginning to come out, can either use gentle cleansing with liquid soap, followed by a cotton ball saturated with **toner** (because of its astringent[1] and aseptic[2] characteristics [i.e. *benzoyl-peroxide*, *tea tree* oil]) then applying a moist warm compress. Or one can use a cotton-swab dipped in **Visine** solution (because of its vasoconstricting[3]/decongesting effect), **Benzoyl-peroxide** (again) or **preparation-H** (a medication for hemorhoids... believe it or not because of its mild cortisone anti-inflammatory effect). Even **over-the-counter (OTC)** topical antibiotic solutions (*erythromycin or cleocin* - if available are effective). One can even try **milk of magnesia or calamine lotion as a facial mask**...for 15 to 20 minutes followed by a rinse. For patients with **itchy-acne or skin itchiness**, another useful **over-the-counter (OTC)** medication, **Sarna solution**, can be used before switching into more powerful and potent topical steroids or cortisone.

III. ENVIRONMENTAL FACTORS

When we talk about environment the things that come to mind are the surrounding temperature, humidity, pollution and even seasons of the year. Although these influences have been found to affect the individual's skin oiliness or dryness, I am going to confine myself to those **acnegenic** or non-comedogenic factors that can affect the individual either directly or indirectly. For instance there are acnes that are triggered by the application of certain cosmetics and thus called **acne cosmetica**. Individuals should be aware of cleansers, toners, make-up or hair formulations that can initiate or trigger acne/pimples.

Industrial acne are those related to exposure to some industrial chemicals while at work in chemical companies that use chlorinated hydrocarbons, coal tar, and even exposure to some printing press copying machine operations where tar is an ingredient of ink. **Frictional or mechanical acne** is the result of **repetitive trauma** which is very common in sports-oriented individuals wearing tight exercise clothing, elastic headbands, elastic bra, belts, abdominal binders and even the frequent and repeated rubbing with sports equipment. **Tropical acne and acne aestivalis** (of summer) have been associated to exposure to hot weather. Treatment consists of changing or moving to a cooler environment. The recent economic crises have triggered a lot of stress resulting in the **increase incidence of acne sufferers in adults**, called **stress acne**.

Some of the more common locations of **acne cosmetica** are the facial or chin areas; pomade (hair-gels and hair styling products) having contact around the forehead and sides of facial areas; toothpaste (fluoride and mentholated) around the mouth area, and telephone receivers frequently touching and rubbing the side of the face (jaw area and chin area) are all frequent stimuli. Even teens blowing bubble gum can start formation of pimples around the mouth. Instead of rushing to the drugstore to buy anti-acne **over-the-counter (OTC)** medications, treatment for **acne cosmetica** can be as simple as identification of the causative agent followed by avoidance of the offending agent(s) or culprit(s). Instead of resting or cradling a phone receiver on the chin and side of the face while talking, a simple solution to avoiding telephone related acne is installation of either a headphone or speakerphone. Basic asepsis/hygiene using handy wipes of various disinfectant gels or solutions could also be applied to the telephone receiver before or after each use. Treatment for **stress-related acne** could be categorized as "better said than done" therapy because of the unpredictability of the problem. They usually affect women who are in sales or high executive positions that travel frequently. It is the pressure of producing sales and making tough decisions, combined with the damaging effects of travel environs that make **stress-related** acne management more challenging.

High stressed-out people supposedly generate an increase of **cortisol, DHT**, and **testosterone**, all of which stimulate the **sebaceous**

oil glands to produce more sebum. This **surge of hormones** along with its subsequent production of more sebum and the added dead cell shedding and pore clogging, induce the proliferation of **p. acnes** and other **bacteria** resulting in **pimple production**.

However, patients should keep in mind that although there is no cure for acne, the complications of acne, such as scarring, pigmentations and **body image changes** can be prevented because these are mostly **self-inflicted** or iatrogenic[1] [induced unintentionally in a patient by the (salon) treatment or by a physician].IF THERE IS NO PICKING, SQUEEZING,SCRATCHING OR INJECTING,THEN THERE SHOULD BE NO PIGMENTATION,INFLAMMATION AND SCARRING.

IV. HORMONAL OR ENDOCRINE DISORDERS

Abnormalities or disease of the endocrine glands /[a gland, such as thyroid, adrenal, or pituitary, having hormonal secretions that pass directly into the bloodstream], particularly the pituitary glands /[this gland has a general controlling power over all the endocrine glands. Lack of the gland's activity shows itself in slow or late sex-development; excess or disorder produces very early sex-development], adrenal glands /[the adrenal gland pours adrenalin into the body when there is sudden fear; this adrenalin causes quicker heart beat, pale skin, etc]. **Polycystic**[1] [containing many cysts] **ovaries**, have been linked to development of acne.

Due to the hormonal influence of these various glands, disorders of these glands, have to be kept in mind when treating stubborn acne. A trial treatment period using less drastic measures has to be tried. If the acne eruptions are recalcitrant or stubborn, these patients may benefit from a complete endocrine work up (necessary laboratory tests) to identify potential underlying causes. Treatment directed towards the cause usually leads to a successful acne therapy.

V. MEDICATIONS: DIFFERENT APPROACHES IN THE TREATMENT OF ACNE

As I mentioned in the previous section, treatment of acne needs to be individualized for it to succeed. **One approach** is to consider such **treatment according to the type of acne causation or offending agents** as in the case of "acne cosmetica". Management consists of identifying the offending sources and treating them accordingly, *by avoidance, *prevention and their *outright elimination. **Another method** is to base the **treatment according to the degree of severity or clinical characteristics**/signs that **the acne patient is currently showing**. This relates to *the number, *the type of acne eruptions, *the presence of inflammation, *pigmentations, *scars and the *potential for more complicated healing such as those with **keloidal tendencies**. These are patients that instead of healing with a flat skin surface, the acne punctured/scratched areas become rough and bumpy. These scars may even continue to grow and become prominent unless properly managed.

What Brings Patients To Our Office?

It is not unusual that patients come to our office because of parents concerned about their children's acne break outs. Very often, we ask our patients the reason why they are in my office, and the retort sometimes is, "I don't know, my mom/dad brought me here!" It is these type of patients, oblivious of their malady, that are subject to treatment failure unless properly educated. These type of patients who are unaware and oblivious, together with those patients who are IN DENIAL, that he or she has a problem, have made the treatment and management of acne formidable and challenging. A patient's acne can never be controlled or more importantly cured, if a person believes that he/she is not sick. Because of the non life threatening nature of acne disease, victims tend to take them for granted until it is too late. There is no amount of doctoring that can help these patients unless they have ACCEPTANCE that a problem exists. It behooves us, physicians, not only to gingerly educate them but firmly caution them that improperly treated or mismanaged acne, although not life threatening, can sometimes lead to disastrous physical and mental consequences. But the frequent and common concerns that bring patients to our office are acne breakouts or inflammation, pigmentation, scarring and psychological **body image** changes.

Types Of Acne According To Clinical Characteristics

Type I or Mild Form of Acne

This is characterized by the presence of a few whiteheads and blackheads, with occasional papules, pustules, approximately 10-15 lesions and associated with absence to mild or minimal pigmentation. The potential for permanent scarring is remote when properly managed.

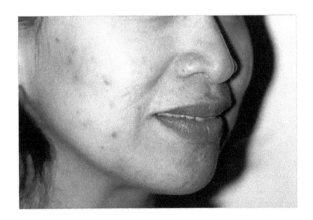

Type I or Mild Form of Acne

Type II or Moderate Form of Acne

This is characterized by the presence of more numerous whiteheads and blackheads, papules, pustules (20 lesions or more) and accompanied with some pigmentations and the possibility of developing superficial to mild scars. The chance of having permanent scar from this type is remote when early diagnosed and treated.

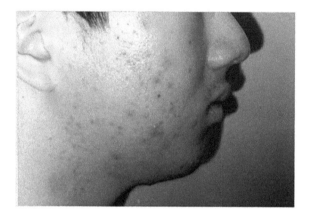

Type II or Moderate Form of Acne

Type III or Severe Form of Acne

Characterized by all of the above findings but in greater number and in various acute and chronic states. These can be in cystic or nodular form often accompanied with pain, pigmentations, inflammation and a very high degree of scarring which could become permanent

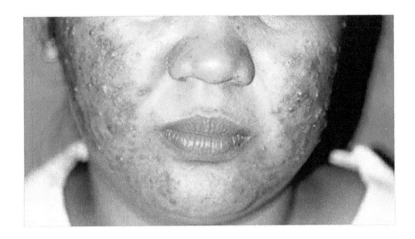

Type III or Severe Form of Acne

In general, most people who suffer from acne DO NOT need to see a dermatologist or a family physician, especially those with Type I and Type II form of acne. With proper education through self-study, most of these acne type problems can be effectively managed with a basic "working knowledge" of skin care gained from self-help books combined with the judicious use of over the counter (OTC) acne medications. Exemptions to this rule are those with a very strong family history of acne, manifested by affliction of both parents and some other siblings. Individuals, particularly bothered psychologically by the appearance of a solitary or group of acne eruptions, and with prior "conventional acne therapy failures" (those non-responsive to **Type I** and **Type II** form of acne cases after few months therapy). I cannot over emphasize THE FACT that IT IS HARD ENOUGH

FOR PHYSICIANS TO MANAGE ACNE, ONE SHOULD SEEK MEDICAL HELP AFTER 3 TO 6 WEEKS OF SLOW AND UNRESPONSIVE SELF MEDICATION. PROGRAM.

Adult Onset Acne (AOA)

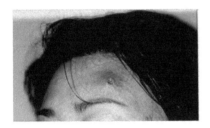 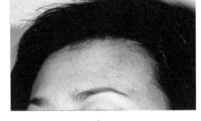

Before   *After*

Just because you are past your teenage and tween years makes one feel immune from the "rite of passage" of the acne phenomenon and its complications. WRONG! Welcome to the world of Adult Onset Acne (AOA) which is reportedly on the rise affecting 50s, 60s and even 70 years old individuals. This is due to a *stress laden environment, *pollution, *hormonal fluctuation and changes in the later year of life, and even plain *improper use of facial creams, lotions and *other rituals. Although **adult onset acne (AOA)** has some genetic predisposition, it is more common in **women (20%)** as compared to **men (8%)**. However, if one is well versed on ways of AcneCx®-Proofing complication prevention then the **incidence of dire acne consequences will be remote**. Hence, a self-help book like this becomes a handy reference for both teenagers and adults.

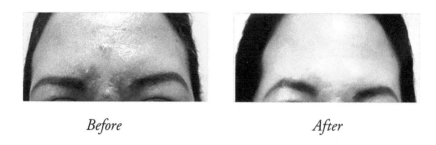

Before   *After*

Successful women in their 50s and 60s having pimples for the first time, is most probably due to the stressful demand of their profession. Incidentally, **there is NO role for local or systemic antibiotic monotherapy in the management of acne.** In other words, by itself, the use of antibiotics on the skin, antibiotics taken by mouth or those given by injection or infusion have NO value or use in the treatment of acne. And while talking about facial break out or infection of the face, allow me to digress on a specific area called:

Dangerous Triangle of the Face

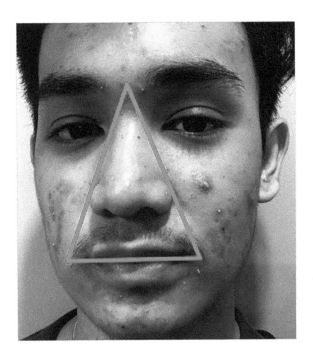

The location of the imaginary **red triangle** (above) is the universally and accepted **dangerous triangle area of the face** by the medical community. This is bounded by two lines from the root of the nose, extending downwards to both corners of the mouth, and going across, just below the free border of the upper lip, to meet the other line. Why is this called the **dangerous triangle of the face**? This is because the blood supply, particularly the venous [full of veins]

portion, are in close proximity to the **brain** and its coverings. Any infection in this area has the potential of spreading to the **brain** or its meninges. Hence, infection in this area, including pimples, have to be treated with the utmost care. Needless to say, **any manipulations, squeezing or massaging of pimples in this area is prohibited as this may lead to brain infection leading to abscess.**

Triple A Principle

A lthough early medical consultation is ideal for facial infection, such is not the case for facial acne if the patient feels confident on self medication. This is only after undergoing a diligent self study for a better understanding of acne, its contributing factors and its complication evolution. And since there is no complete cure of acne, the main focus of therapy should be on minimizing or totally preventing acne complications. These complications can be in the form of pigmentations, scars, psychological overlays and low self-esteem. Unfortunately, these consultations will require a caring, **empathetic** and knowledgeable physician, and not just some doctor who performs a hasty examination followed by prescriptions of their favorite anti-acne medications. Patients today are mostly educated and they should not hesitate to ask their doctors on matters which are not clear and understandable to them. Should there be any doubt; a second opinion from another physician may be in order. As I have alluded earlier, patients equipped with a working knowledge of his/her problem, particularly the rationale of the recommended treatment program and its compliance very often lead to a successful outcome.

In addition to learning the pathophysiology or mechanism of how these acne complications develop, for acne therapy to succeed, whether physician directed or through self-medication, one has to have these three important considerations and facts in mind:

a) AWARENESS OR ACCEPTANCE of the disease,
b) its ANALYSIS,
c) and its immediate ACTION.

This is called **THE TRIPLE "A" PRINCIPLE** and these are the factors that have to be kept in mind especially for those on self-medication.

AWARENESS OR ACCEPTANCE means the patient has to be aware and accepts that he/she has an acne problem. Oftentimes, patients are in denial. Unless he is aware and accepts that he has an acne problem, then there is nothing to treat. NO physician can treat an illness that the patient believes does not exist. However, once he has awareness and acceptance of his skin situation, the next step is to:

ANALYZE AND EVALUATE the problem by trying to determine and understand the possible causes especially those that are preventable and correctable as previously and subsequently described in some parts of this book. Special attention on the clinical characteristics, risk factors, the degree of severity of the person's acne problem and the potential for severe and permanent acne scarring should be made. Based on these analyses a treatment protocol and its options can be designed accordingly. A treatment program based on these analyses can then be designed accordingly.

ACTION ON THE ACTION PLAN means the immediate implementation and strict compliance to the designed treatment program is mandatory. With complications prevention as the main focus of the treatment, the immediate identification and stoppage of any obvious harmful habits such as pimple popping, squeezing, massaging, etc have to be done with an empathetic WHY explanation and the subsequent dire consequences if such habits are not aborted or stopped. This act alone can show visible and measurable effect usually in a matter of few days or even less. These alone can show visible and measurable effect instantly or a a matter of few days. No matter how good a regimen is, in the end the treatment plan, **unless acted upon,** boils down to nothing. With the skyrocketting cost of HEALTHCARE all over the world, particularly, the pharmaceuticals, more and more health providers are encouraging the use of preventative measures, thus, the participation and cooperation of patients are paramount. This is why strict compliance is absolutely essential and should be the concern of both the patient and the treating physician. This is even more applicable in treating acne, which is a very common and a seemingly harmless skin disease but with devastating consequences and complications if left untreated or mismanaged. There should be close monitoring of the treatment program and its progress once it has commenced.

Combining this **TRIPLE "A" PRINCIPLE of a) AWARENESS/ACCEPTANCE, b) ANALYSIS, and c) ACTION,** and **an a treatment paradigm shift from Acne cure to Acne complications prevention, Type I or mild form of acne** and **Type II or moderate form of acne** can usually be treated effectively even without a physician's assistance. You do have to be a **DISCERNING, AVID, AND VORACIOUS** label reader in seeking the **BEST** and **SAFEST over-the-counter (OTC)** medicine or home remedy type of medications for your acne. These should include learning about the main ingredients, indications (how they work), contraindications, and most importantly, instructions on its proper applications and use. A limited period of self medication of a few weeks may be tried if the patient feels confident using **over-the-counter (OTC)** medicines and home remedies. However, should there be any doubt in his/her mind, a proper medical consultation with a family physician/dermatologist should be made. I could not over emphasize enough to learn and master the mechanism of mild to moderate acne complication evolution because it is in these types I and II that permanent complications like pigmentation and scarring can be prevented with AcneC$^{\circledR}_x$-Proofing protocol.

ALL Type III or Severe Form of Acne should ONLY BE TREATED BY DERMATOLOGISTS or BY PHYSICIANS "on-the-know". With these principles, together with a paradigm/attitude shift in the treatment objective of complications prevention instead of cure, let us begin acne management based on the type/classification of acne according to its clinical characteristics.

Treatment of Acne According to Clinical Characteristics

TYPE I or MILD FORM OF ACNE is characterized by a few whiteheads, blackheads, papules and pustules with very minimal to NO chance of scarring or pigmentations. Please bear in mind that these **blackheads are NOT DIRT**. Scrubbing or rubbing does not make the skin any cleaner or smoother but, on the contrary, might stimulate the already sensitive sebaceous/oil gland resulting in the production of more oil. As long as there is NO **pricking**, **squeezing**, **scratching** or any mechanical **abrasive** manipulation, no pigmentation or scarring should ensue. ACTION course on this might just be a basic **GENTLE, non-vigorous washing** routine such as foaming gels or enzyme based detergents. **Avoid bar soaps because the ingredient that makes the soap solid is comedogenic.** If within 28 to 45 days no improvement is noted, start a mildest **over-the-counter (OTC)** or non prescription medication(s) (mild exfoliants, disinfectants for oily skin type: **Benzoyl peroxide**, **Salicylic acid**, **glycolic acids**, etc) for 3 to 6 weeks. If there is still minimal to no response, then a higher strength **over-the-counter (OTC)** medication or more aggressive form of treatment has to be implemented. In the United States, and other parts of the world pharmacists and nurse practitioners are legally allowed to suggest and recommend **over-the-counter (OTC)** and even certain prescription medications. Such an inquiry might not only be valuable but also cost effective. However, IF the patient does not feel comfortable self-medicating using **over-the-counter (OTC)** or home remedy approaches, then an early medical consultation should be sought. The old adage that "an ounce of prevention is better than a pound of cure", is pertinent in this situation.

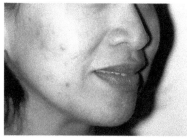
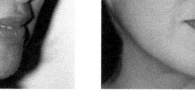

Before   After

~

TYPE II or MODERATE FORM OF ACNE is characterized by more numerous papules, pustules and comedones, accompanied by some pigmentations and potential risks of scarring. This form of acne should be still be managable with **over-the-counter (OTC)** or non-prescription medications as described in Type I. However, to expedite or obtain faster response, using stronger strength exfoliants combined with various prescription medications (**retinoids** and **antibiotics**) may have to be started. Management of the Type II form of acne is done with the full understanding of the contributing factors and potential complications in mind.

These complications may range in various degrees of pigmentations and scarring, all of which are preventable since most of them are **self-inflicted**. If there is no **pricking**, **squeezing** or any **scratching**, then no scarring or pigmentation will arise. A specific therapeutic period of 28 to 45 days has to be designated to evaluate the effect or non-effect of the regimen used. Should there be any doubt or reservations as to the patient's capabilities to a self-medication program, then a medical consultation should be obtained. ACTION course consists of gentle cleansers, exfoliants, **retinoids**, in combination with oral or topical **antibiotics** should stronger **over-the-counter (OTC)** medications have no effect.

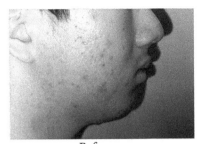 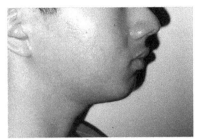

Before	After

TYPE III or SEVERE FORM OF ACNE is characterized by the appearance of more numerous (more than 10) cystic and nodular lesions in addition to comedones, papules and pustules. Some of these have abscesses with associated pain, pigmentation and various stages of scarring. Patients also show signs of frustration and depression, low esteem, and other body image problems which may result in a curtailed life-style of self-imposed social exile. **TREATMENT OF TYPE III ACNE IS RESERVED ONLY FOR DERMATOLOGISTS AND PHYSICIANS** "on-the-know". The help of other medical specialists (psychiatrist, endocrinologist, gynecologist, etc) may be needed. Physicians have to quickly determine the risk factors and possible triggers, which when identified can be eliminated/avoided. A prescribed treatment program is usually a combination of **exfoliants, antibiotics, retinoids** and **counseling**. It is also during this time that we introduce **meditation** (prayer) with **creative visualization**. This is supplemented by verbal positive affirmations. Although treatment is usually successful in controlling acne, complications such as scarring and pigmentations are quite common.

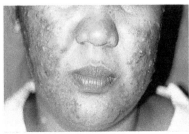 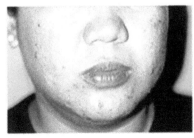

Before	After

This is why, for those suffering from acne,

Acne in any type or form is STILL Acne. EARLY DIAGNOSIS AND TREATMENT IS IMPERATIVE combined with a laser focused goal of COMPLICATIONS PREVENTION not cure. Departing from such goal may lead to severe and perhaps a lifetime of miseries and regrets. THINK PREVENTION NOT CURE!

Universality of Acne

IT OCCURS NOW IN ALL AGES!
OCCURS IN ALL NATIONS
- **WHETHER RICH OR POOR,**
- **INDUSTRIALIZED**
- **UNDERDEVELOPED**
- **OR THIRD WORLD NATIONS**

Sobering statistics: 650 million acne cases worldwide and the direct cost of the disease exceeds U.S.$3 Billion per year. Despite the information bombardment on the public about the latest treatment of acne, especially those of the wealthy industrialized nations, acne and its complications remain high. In fact, the **incidence** of **adult onset acne (AOA)** has actually **increased**. According to a recent study in the American Academy of Dermatology Journal, 53% of women over the age of 33 have acne. "It is certainly a lot more common than it was 100 years ago," says Dr. Richard Glogau, a professor of Dermatology at the University of California, San Francisco. Hence, acne is no longer a teenage phenomenon alone but also increasingly found in adulthood. Teenagers of these wealthy industrialized countries are probably the most familiar with the latest acne treatments, as they are the targeted audience. We advise caution on these "infomercials" as some may contain "half-truths" and are outright misleading. These "infomercials" (especially print, radio-broadcast and television), are not necessarily the most knowledgeable as far as home remedies and proper **over-the-counter (OTC)** anti-acne medications are concerned. Let us all be an educated, discerning and discriminating consumer.

Take note that if acne remains common in the presumably more educated, wealthy, industrialized countries, it becomes even more important for poor third world / undeveloped countries to familiarize and learn for themselves as many preventive measures of acne complications as they can. They must educate themselves on the proper use of established **over-the-counter (OTC)** acne medicines or home remedies. When properly administered, such knowledge might be helpful and cost-effective, since they are usually cheaper than prescription medications.

Before discussing **over-the-counter (OTC)** drug or home remedy medications let me mention a very annoying and common accompanying symptom in patients with acne, which is **excessive facial "oiliness or sweating".** This facial oiliness may actually be present even in the absence of acne eruptions. The causative mechanism of this condition is unknown, hence the treatment is symptomatic and empirical at best. Some oil absorbing paper, powders, creams and gels from various compositions of astringents, acrylic polymers and silica maybe located under the name **Clinac, Seban** and **Neova.**

What Is an Over-the-Counter (OTC) Drug or Home Remedy Medication?

These are non-prescription drugs that have undergone the necessary screening as to their EFFECTIVITY and SAFETY required by the **FOOD and DRUG ADMINISTRATION (FDA)** of the individual country, using United States methodology as the gold standard or model for such screening procedures. Approval can be found in the form of a seal or coded number. It is right and fitting that the public not only be discerning but also be an informed and be an educated consumer if he or she were to expect a successful result, utilizing **over-the-counter (OTC)** drugs. One has to be an avid label reader and follow specific instructions in order to achieve optimum outcome.

What makes a drug classified as **over-the-counter (OTC)** is often based on the strength or concentration of the main active ingredient. It is not unusual for an **over-the-counter (OTC)** drug to have various ranges of concentration or strength. For first time users, after doing your diligent research, inquiring from your local or neighborhood pharmacist might be your initial move. Otherwise we advise using the lowest effective recommended concentration or strength when doing self-medication. Among the common **over-the-counter (OTC)** anti-acne medications are the following:

EXFOLIANT: KERATOLYTIC or DESQUAMATING/ (peel-off) AGENT are topically applied formulations in the form of liquid, cream, or gel that loosens the top layer cells of the outer skin and the lining of the **follicular canal**. Because of this loosening/unclogging effect, the plugs that are formed in the **pores are decongested and unblocked decreasing the incidence of acne formation**. Regardless of volume production of sebum/oil, as long as there is unobstructed flow to the outer skin, the chance of developing acne is minimized if not prevented. This is why the judicious/(sensible, proper) use of **exfoliants** alone or in combination with other drugs, can be quite effective in treating acne. **Benzoyl peroxide (BPO)** at 2% to 10% is probably the most popular **over-the-counter** anti-acne drug, because it is both an **exfoliant** and a disinfectant. **BPO's** disinfectant and antibacterial action against **p.acnes** and other **anaerobic bacteria** present in the **follicular canal** thus eliminate the immediate need for antibiotics sometimes required in more challenging acne cases. **Alpha hydroxy acids (AHA) (glycolic acid** 1% to 8%, **lactic acid** 1% to 5%) are also effective **exfoliants** but not as effective as the **beta hydroxy acids (BHA) salicylic acid** (0.5% to 2%) as far as exfoliation is concerned. **BHA salicylic acid**, because of its being soluble in oil has been proven effective in the treatment of acne as compared to **AHAs**. Its lack of antibacterial activity against **p.acnes**, the most common offending acne agent required its combination with **BPO** or other antibacterial drugs. **Resorcinol** 2% to 3% and **sulfur** 3% to 8% are both **exfoliants** and antibacterial. Low strength **tretinoine** 0.025% have also been used as **over-the-counter exfoliants**. The flaking or peeling effect of these **exfoliants** require strict sun protection compliance. It is therefore IMPERATIVE that the direction of use and proper application of **sunscreen** MUST BE OBSERVED. A more detailed dissertation on this very important and vital subject is covered at a later chapter.

For **Type I and Type II acne**, along with the careful use of the above **exfoliants**, together with a working knowledge of how acne develops, the awareness and understanding of the risks factors, avoidance of potential causes, and a tempered/balanced emotional concern of the disease, one can expect a visual and satisfactory outcome.

ANTIBIOTICS are drugs that are used to kill **bacteria**. Systemic or local antibiotics, ALONE, have NO role in acne therapy or acne control. They have to be used in combination with other modalities of treatment either to prevent or treat developing or existing infection. We have to remember that the normally inhabiting **p. acnes** and other anaerobic **bacteria** only causes inflammation when there is blockage and the lining integrity of the **follicular canal** has been disrupted. This allows **bacteria** to invade deeper tissues. This is usually triggered by induced manipulations of picking, **squeezing**, pricking or even scrubbing. **Antibiotics** can be oral or topical and require medical prescription, hence a medical consultation. This has to be done when there is any doubt as to the patient's ability to self-administer standard anti-acne regimen. A few weeks trial period of **over-the-counter (OTC)** drug treatment may be indicated. Initially we advised the use of topical **antibiotics** in gel, cream, or solution instead of oral route. This treatment is not only directed precisely on the areas of concern but also give us better control of complications, should they arise. The more popular **topical antibiotics** (usually according to physician's preference) are: **erythromycin** in alcohol solution or ointment, and **clindamycin** also in its variety or preparations. These can be applied once or twice a day. Among the commonly used **oral antibiotics** for acne is **tetracycline**. This should be taken an hour or two before each meal. Children under the age of 10 years, **lactating or pregnant women should NOT take** this since it can cause some dental staining of their babies. **Clindamycin, erythromycin, doxycycline,** and **minocycline** are other **antibiotics** that have been found to be effective for acne. CAUTION: oral antibiotics may cause some gastrointestinal distress in the form of nausea, vomiting, or diarrhea. **Monilia or yeast infection** of the genital tract is not uncommon in individuals taking oral **antibiotics**. Needless to say, using antibiotics have to be under physician's supervision and direction.

TRETINOINE OR RETINOIC ACID is a **vitamin A derivative** that is probably the most effective drug being used to eliminate or control acne, with **tretinoine 0.025% to 0.1%** as its signature product. Its action is based on reduction of oil/sebum production and the loosening of the dead cells that are clogging up the lining of the **follicular canal** and outer skin. These are two important contributing factors in the development of acne eruptions. Because of **Tretinoine**'s drying, and peeling off effects on the skin, pores are unclogged. Accompanying local reactions are sometimes severe, hence its use is better under medical supervision. Recent improvements of **tretinoine** have lessened their side effects and made them more effective and tolerable. This can be applied once or twice a day depending on the strength or concentration of the drug. Other **tretinoine-like** drugs include **azelaic acid (Azelex)** which acts as: (1) keratolytic, (2) bactericidal, and (3) an added bleaching effect needed for the pigmentation that usually accompanies **Type II** and **Type III** acne. **Azelaic acid** can therefore become the ideal topical treatment for acne because of this triple effect. **Differin** and **Tazorac** are the other prescription medications found to be effective in the management of acne because of their keratolytic action. CAUTION: All these drugs are prescription medications and should not be used in pregnant women. The use of sunblock or sunscreen during the day is mandatory.

ACCUTANE or **13-CIS-RETINOIC ACID** or **ISOTRETINOINE** is a synthetic **derivative of vitamin A**, and is sometimes labeled as the "miracle or magic drug" for acne because of its sometimes dramatic effect on the severest form of cystic acne. It is a very powerful and strong oral medication that has to be handled with utmost care; and deliberation/(caution) especially in women of childbearing age. Reports **linking Accutane to birth defects** in babies born to mothers who were taking the drug, and **incidence of suicide** by the individuals taking the same have been reported. Due to the obvious gravity of these potential outcomes, a full, detailed discussion of the program together with its expected reactions, risks, and potential complications, need to be done by the doctor, patient and a responsible relative. This is followed by a written and signed consent allowing the treating physician to administer the program. Before starting treatment on this drug, which is taken 16 to 20 weeks, the patient before usage needs to take a battery of tests consisting of the following: 1) complete blood count, 2) chemical and liver profile, with 3) monthly rechecking of albumin[1], cholesterol[2] and triglyceride[3] levels. Follow-up laboratory results allow physicians to alter subsequent dosages. The use of this drug seems formidable, discouraging, and prohibitive. But, a properly administered program on a fully informed patient with severe cystic acne disease not only results in the control of the disease but sometimes cures the cystic acne. This may require one or two therapeutic cycles at 6 to 8 weeks interval. **Other reactions or side effects of Accutane of lesser gravity** are the over all drying effect of not only the skin but also all the mucous membrane lined cavities such as the mouth, eyes nose, urethra (genital areas) and anal area. Hence, adequate use of moisturizers and liberal oral intake of water (Note: excluding sodas and liquor) can alleviate the discomfort. Precaution: Headaches, dizziness, and blurring of vision have also been reported.

Quick Reference	
Benzoyl Peroxide	Antibacterial
Salicylic Acid	Exfoliate,
Glycolic Acid	Exfoliate
Tretinoine	Reduce sebum/oil
Azelaic Acid	Blends & reduce oil
Tea Tree	Cleanse, heals
Green Tea	Antioxidant, heals
Licorice	Brightener & blend
Papaya	Brightener
Minocycline	Antibiotic
Kojic Acid	Whitening
Hydroquinone	Whitening
Melfade	Brightener, blend
Erythromycin	Antibiotic

A reduction in dosage usually helps in the relief of these symptoms. With the possibility of these significant reactions and side effects, I cannot over emphasize the importance of warning patients of the possible appearance of these reactions that are sometimes mistakenly considered as allergic reactions. **CAUTION: WOMEN TAKING ACCUTANE SHOULD BE ON A FOOLPROOF CONTRACEPTION REGIMEN**, bearing in mind that use of **antibiotics** may alter the effects of birth control pills.

When Can a Woman Plan for Conception after Using Accutane to Avoid Birth Defects?

It has been reported that a two to three-month cessation from the use of **Accutane** has not increased the incidence of birth defect(s) on newborns.

Acne and the Birth Control Pill

Birth Control Pills are **hormonal drugs** that either lower the testosterone level *per se* or block the oil producing effect of testosterone, thus **minimizing the incidence of acne**. Although **Ortho Tri-Cyclen** was the first FDA approved birth control pill for acne use, other oral contraceptives like **Desogen, Alesse, Yasmin**, and **Ortho-Cept** have a similar effect. There are some high-progestin pills that can actually exacerbate acne eruption. Hence, a woman with acne who is simultaneously seeking **oral contraception** would be served best by a consultation with her obstetrician-gynecologist.

What Can We Do with the Increase Acne Eruptions a Week Prior to or during Menstrual Period

Women are often advised about the increased **hormonal (testosterone) surge** during menstruation resulting in the increase of acne breakouts. There is not much anyone can do but to "let the cycle take its course." This seemingly hopeless and helpless feeling only contributes and exacerbates the patient's already stress laden condition, thus aggravating and triggering more acne eruptions.

In our practice, if the birth control pills under obstetrician/gynecologist guidance fails, we found the combination of **over-the-counter retinoids** and **exfoliants** to be effective and quite beneficial both psychologically and physiologically. Mindful of the unclogging effect and the reduced oil production of the **retinoid/exfoliant (RET-EX)** combination, it has been our experience that such combination, at proper dosage, has been adequate to counteract the unwelcome increase of pimple appearance due to **hormonal surge** during menstruation. This unexpected but pleasant decrease in acne breakouts produced cosmetically pleasing changes on the face. These cosmetic facial improvements, noticeable by both the patient and treating physician, are significant and important observations. It is the increase appearance of acne eruptions prior to or during menstrual period which is a common and major cause of STRESS.

The MORE STRESS, the MORE ACNE BREAKOUTS!

Taking some COMPASSIONATE time to explain the importance of "HOW" and "WHY" there is a stress-reduction EFFECT of **Tretinoine** and **exfoliants** to acne sufferers have paid dividends to our patients. Such physiological unclogging of the pores through **exfoliation** and the **retinoid** driven sebum reduction are added benefits of such combination.

Hence, when patients experience an increase in acne eruptions during or one week prior to their menstruation, they now have a solution to rely on, instead of helplessly "allowing nature's cycle to take its course." Therefore, an **OTC retinoid** cream or gel may become handy. A more proactive use of the **retinoid/exfoliant** regimen a few days prior to their menstrual cycle has decreased patient's fear and stress of ugly uncontrollable acne eruptions.

In Search of a Model: Consistently Effective and with a Universal Approach to Acne

Dr. Debra Jaliman, a New York dermatologist and spokesperson for the American Academy of Dermatology, was quoted recently that regardless of the cause and severity of acne, treatment has never been more plentiful and effective. She added that acne sufferers today are actually luckier to be born in this day and age because of all these recent advances in acne therapy.

The question most frequently asked is:

If indeed, we are at a cutting edge era of acne therapy . . .

Why is the Incidence of Acne Increasing in Both Teenagers and Adults?

I believe that it is partly because for the past 50 to 70 years most teenagers and lots of adults were totally ignorant and remained uneducated or misinformed on the evolution of acne, its diagnosis, management, and its complications. Except for a few sentences, medical textbooks, journals and magazines, information is found wanting and glaringly **LACKED PROACTIVE topics of ACNE COMPLICATIONS PREVENTION**. MITIGATING therapy has been focused on symptomatic "quick-fix Band-aid˚ type treatments" frequently resulting in short-term gratification and improvements, but oftentimes, with disastrous results. Self-manipulations on acne, by the patient or at a salon or doctor's clinic, remain a very common self-destructive ritual. More aggressive emphasis on education, counseling, and preventive methods of acne complications, should be the primary focus. This will certainly supplement the improvement that acne chemically derived products bring. It is only by educating and making the public aware of the dire consequences of untreated/ mismanaged acne that complications can be minimized and in some cases prevented. I submit that most if not all of these acne complications are preventable if the individual follows a certain protocol with heavy emphasis on prevention!

How Do We Manage Itching on Acne Patients?

Although acne/pimple per se is not accompanied by **itching**, a lot of the acne medications both prescriptive and non-prescriptive type are oftentimes associated with **itching**. This is particularly true for those keratolytic, desquamating, exfoliating or "peeling" lotions and creams.

Itching, unless properly addressed, may actually aggravate the clinical features of acne by predisposing it to the development of scarring and pigmentations. These are the complications of acne that are totally avoidable and preventable. To do this, one has to consider **itching** as similar to pain sensation. It is a sensory symptom or stimulus that starts from the skin passing through a nerve pathway and ending up in the brain's itch OR pain center where it is interpreted as an itch OR pain stimulus. In our office we have been successful in avoiding or minimizing the effects of **scratching** (ie pigmentation and scarring) by disrupting and breaking the usual straight forward pattern of the sensory nerve pathway from the skin to the brain center. **Scratching**, the usual automatic or reflex response to our body's itch sensation, can be stopped or aborted when patients are instructed of the following: a) conscious tapping or snapping with the hand, finger or blunt instrument over the itchy area; b) cold compress application with the use of ice cubes/bags, air condition or electric fan; c) topical anesthetic application; d) topical antihistaminic or cortisone medications; and e) picker pincher stopper application. All these actions will not result in scars or **hyper pigmentation** as compared to the **reflex scratching** which causes excoriation and abrasions of the affected area leading to unnecessary scarring and pigmentations. By disrupting and interrupting the itch sensory pathway with a non-traumatic stimulus such as tapping or sudden application of cold compress, the urge to scratch is markedly diminished. These actions lessen the chance of scarring and pigmentation from **scratching**. After a few days of using one of these maneuvers, the body develops tolerance leading to less itchiness even with their continued use.

Can Acne Scarring, Pigmentation, Low Self-Esteem, Anger, Frustrations, Problems Related to Body Image, and in Severe Cases, Suicide, be Prevented or Minimized?

The answer to this question is a: **"BIG YES"**! This is proven by the hundreds of acne patients we have successfully treated in the past 30 to 35 years in our medical practice. How does our corrESthetiques®Way AcneCx®-Proofing Program differ from the currently accepted and practiced acne regimen? The primary difference is that our **ADDED EMPHASIS OF THERAPY is directed on PREVENTION OF THE TWO MOST VISUAL AND NOTICEABLE COMPLICATIONS OF ACNE, WHICH ARE SCARRING AND PIGMENTATIONS COMBINED WITH MENTAL CALISTHENICS, POWERED BY A GOAL SETTING WHAT-HOW-WHY (WHW) SYSTEM.**

We now live in a "looks oriented society". Unfortunately, we are judged according to "how our faces look". This becomes even more important on acne prone people since the acne disease starts seemingly harmless. Facial eruptions later develop into full-blown physical and emotional scarring with sometimes disastrous and devastating effects. The CONCERN for the development of **facial scarring** and secondary pigmentations are what make acne patients go for their first office visit. These patients are given early preventive "how to" instructions, emphasizing that acne scars and pigmentations can be avoided or minimized. This should lead to reduced incidence of low-self esteem and **body image problems**. As stated earlier, there is not much anybody can do about the **excessive oil production** and the **excessive peeling off** or **desquamation** of the skin's top layer and lining of the **follicular canal**. This genetic trait, one of the major contributory factors, in combination with the **clogging of the pores and bacterial invasion lead to acne formation**. Such occurrence is inevitable and there is nothing anybody can do.

Acne facial scarring and pigmentation, on the other hand, are the result of: **self-inflicted injury** or **improperly trained and misguided salon technicians or clinic induced injury through squeezing** (comedo whitehead/blackhead extraction), **pricking, scrubbing, or even just stroking the skin**. These self-inducing skin manipulations are obviously stoppable and preventable. Logically, if there is no injury (even as simple as a scratch/abrasion or a puncture) then no scar will follow.

The pigmentations that accompany acne scarring are usually the result of hemoglobin breakdown and degradation following trauma and the ensuing inflammation. The red colored hemoglobin gets reduced to the brown colored **hemosiderin**. If the injury is recurrent and chronic then the discoloration becomes darker and deeper. In the absence of skin injury or trauma, it is obvious that no pigmentation or discoloration will appear.

Most psychological symptoms from acne, like low self-esteem and **body image problems** are the result of the deforming **facial scars** and associated **pigmentations**. Teaching them how to prevent or minimize these scars will certainly result in a healthier, smoother, radiant facial skin and a stable, robust physical and mental state.

How Do We Accomplish this Primary Goal of Scar Avoidance?

First and foremost, there has to be an ACCEPTANCE AND REALIZATION by the affected individual of his/her problematic skin acne. If the individual is just acne prone by reason of genetics and does not have the full blown clinical signs of acne we counsel them at length on how acne scar and pigmentations develop, with emphasis of its potential physical and psychological complications and our suggested proven remedies. Because these complications are mostly **SELF-INFLICTED** procedures or services commonly done in beauty salons and even medical clinics, these can be totally discontinued, thus avoiding these complications. For patients in denial of their condition and who refuse to learn preventive measures to avoid facial scarring, pigmentation and its **psychological overlay**, it is almost tantamount to committing COSMETIC/PSYCHOLOGICAL SELF-SABOTAGE (suicide). Unless he/she actively and consciously participates in the strict compliance of his/her acne management, including, counseling on what they can and cannot do, treatment will certainly fail. Therapeutic success in these cases rely primarily on patients having informed and educated CHOICES. Such decision depends on how badly the patient wants to control and get rid of their potential disfiguring acne complications.

Avoidance of "The Automatic Squeezing" or Reflex "Popping" of Pimples?

Squeezing or **popping pimples** is probably the most common form of **self-inflicted** skin injury that an acne patient first experiences. It is done with the mistaken belief of ridding oneself of infection or dirt.

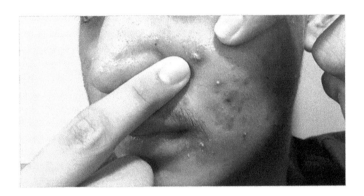

Unfortunately, this seemingly harmless maneuver is accompanied not only by a feeling of self-satisfaction/gratification and well-being but sometimes a great feeling of euphoria. The very sight of this whitish sebum exudate due to squeezing causes patients so much pleasure. Very often this leads to habit formation, to the point of being an **"automatic or reflex"** behavior or mannerism. It is not unusual that because these patients have been used to "**popping**" these pimples for sometime, that they are not even aware that they are **popping** them. This terrible repetitive habit has to be broken and stopped because this will lead to infection, inflammation, pigmentation, scarring, deformity, and subsequent **psychological body image problems**.

Utilizing a psychiatric principle of substitution in breaking up a bad habit, which in this case "popping and squeezing, we advise our 3rd world patients to obtain a portion of orange/lemon skin/ peel and squeeze it hard intermittently. Such action would emit not only a gel like exudate but also a very pleasant smelling orange aroma.

Altho this will not eliminate the squeezing and pricking habit that we encourage to stop, such maneuver have helped some patients relieve their stress related acne issues. Recently, what may seem to be a "whacky solution for a whacky medical issue like acne" the attention of one of TV Shark Tank's investors ventured thousands of dollars into "POPITPAL stress relieving toy. Bear in mind that habitual squeezing, massaging or any type of stimulation of any gland or muscle can lead to hypertrophy or enlargement. Doing the exact opposite principle causes atrophy or loss of bulk. Hence the common adage "if you don't use it, you lose it!" A well recognized and proven physiologic principle. By analogy using the orange skin and the POPITPAL toy as a substitute for your own skin to squeeze, on long term "pimple poppers/squeezers" may be of help in breaking this seemingly innocuous but harmful habit of acne patients.

We address and clarify these issues at the first office visit. Detailed medical history, physical examination, diagnosis and treatment options are discussed including properly authorized photos of the patients. We make the habit of taking before and after pictures of all our patients. Taking authorized close-up facial photos is MANDATORY in my practice as this is our only way of monitoring the patient's actual progress. This is where smartphone selfies, Facetime and Zooming become very handy not only in diagnosing, treating and following the progress of patients. This is specially useful on remote patients. Observing the improvement with actual photographs taken prior and after weeks of therapy not only give the physician an excellent way of monitoring and following the patient's progress but it is also for the patient's own interest. Indirectly, such photos become a yardstick of the patient's proper compliance or non compliance of the treatment program. Providing patients copies of their "before and after" photos helped minimize their chance of going back to their old harmful habits. We encourage our patients to utilize the before and after photographs as vivid/clear reminders of their acne related past imperfections. In the early phase of therapy, some mount their picture in their bathroom vanity, wallet, bracelet or locket. The idea is to remind them of the humiliating and unattractive consequences of mismanaged or untreated acne. Hopefully, this should incentivize them against going back to their old misguided destructive facial habit and rituals.

Having convinced and enlightened patients that **self-induced trauma** (picking, **squeezing**, **popping**, even stroking, etc) is a **major contributing factor in the development of acne scars and pigmentations**, we designed a "**Squeezer, Picker-Pincher Stopper**" sticker applied to the pulp or soft "pinching surface" of the thumb and the index (pointer) fingers. Or, they may use commonly available stickers with smooth surfaces with various religious, positive affirmations and even comedic funny faces, as shown below.

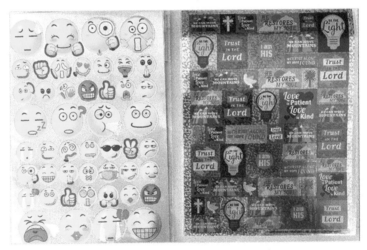

(courtesy Greenbrier International, Inc).

Use of the smooth surfaced stickers together with repeated positive affirmations, not only prevented the urge to reflex picking or pricking but also have secondarily taught our patients some type of discipline in breaking a bad habit with potential disastrous results. This method has been most effective if done continuously for at least 21 days as most new habits are formed or broken in 21 days. To recap: Cleanse both index fingers, thumbs and keep dry. Apply stickers on both opposing surfaces of thumb and index finger daily for 21 days. Reapply when needed. These stickers should be **reminders for acne**

patients not to stroke, massage, prick or **squeeze any pimple** or nodulations of the face.

It is not unusual for someone to slip from the rigid, deliberate and conscious effort of acne treatment, such as **"occasional reflex popping or squeezing of pimples"**. The patient should not be hard on oneself because of the occasional slip. As soon as the patient is **AWARE** of their slippage, they should immediately **STOP SQUEEZING or POPPING** and start doing **SLOW, DEEP-BREATHING EXERCISE**. This should be **repeated six or seven times**, consciously feeling the air as it goes into the air passages **(nostrils) as one inhales**; and then, feeling the air coming out of the lungs, through the air passages and **out of the mouth as one exhales** as in a sigh. This maneuver is even **more effective if creative, positive visualization and imaging accompanies this breathing method**. In other words, one has to picture in one's mind the slow "in and out" flow of air as one inhales through the nose and exhales through the mouth as if he/she were to feel and visualize the movement of the air as it flows and passes through the various air passages. As long as the patient keeps in mind that **it takes repetitive trauma to develop significant scarring and pigmentation** then future and permanent disfiguring scars or pigmentations will no longer develop with the strict compliance of his/her prescribed acne treatment regimen. Behavioral scientists have found VERBAL positive affirmations can augment in achieving one's goal.

Pigmentation in Acne Patients

How is it Developed and What can be Done About Them?

When we talk about the causative factors of pigmentation, the culprits are: 1) sun exposure, 2) hormonal influence, and 3) genetics. It is obvious that there is not much one can do about hormones and genetics. However, we can certainly do something to avoid, if not minimize, the effect of unprotected sun exposure. This can only be achieved by proper use of sunblock. If there is another important lesson gained from reading this book, it would be knowing and understanding the proper use of **sunblock or sunscreen**.

Sunblocks/Sunscreens

It is a fact that the **sun** is the number one **cause of pigmentations**! It is also the number one **cause of wrinkles** and the number one **cause of sun-related skin cancer**. One will never go wrong in learning the what, when, and how **sunblock or sunscreens** are properly applied. Regardless of which part of the globe you come from, the

most harmful time for an individual to be exposed to the sun is during midday or **12 o'clock noon**. This is the time of the day that a person needs sun protection most. A crude guide on when to use **sunblock** is by looking at your shadow. The less shadow you see, the more **sunblock** you should use. However, to play it safe, especially if it is cloudy outside, the **BEST way to protect** yourself against the harmful effects of the sun is to **apply sunblock/sunscreen** at **9 AM** and **mandatory repeated at 12 Noon**. This has to be applied daily, whether you are in the house, office or in your car, rain or shine. For simplicity sake, there are two main types of **sunblock**. The physical blocker which can be applied immediately and provides immediate protection, represented by **titanium oxide** and **zinc oxide**. The other type is the chemical **sunblock** which requires a "reaction time" of 20 to 30 minutes to react with the skin to provide the individual the proper sun shield. The **minimum sun protection factor (SPF)** required is **SPF 15**. Regardless of SPF value, **ALL sunblocks last 1 to 2 hours**. Hence it is suggested that **sunblocks** should **be applied every 2 hours** or even more often, if swimming or playing under a scorching sun. It is better to apply more **sunblock** frequently, rather than have your protection based on a high SPF. Make sure that your **sunblock** protects you from harmful effects of both **UVA** and **UVB** rays of the sun. For better sun protection, DEPEND MORE ON THE FREQUENCY OF APPLICATIONS RATHER THAN THE **SUNBLOCK**'S HIGH SPF.

There is no strict international standard on **sunscreen** dosage specifics, although a 2mg/cm sq have been suggested. A simpler and closer agreement between the expected and delivered **sunscreen** protection is doing the **"finger tip" method**. This entails the application of a strip of **sunscreen** cream or gel from the distal crease of one's index finger to the tip. (See Photo).

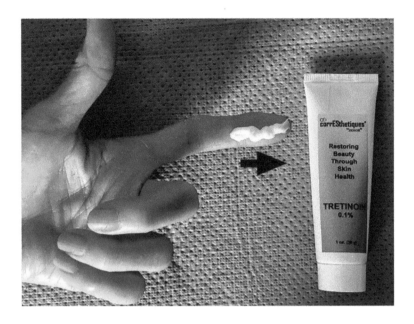

Repetitiveness or Chronicity of Trauma or Injury

Another causative pigmentary factor that is underestimated if not ignored is: REPETITIVENESS or CHRONICITY of TRAUMA or INJURY. This becomes important in dark complexioned individuals with acne because their pigmentation is more pronounced due to the presence of a larger number of **melanocytes** *[a (dark) pigment-producing cell located in the basal layer of the epidermis with branching processes by means of which melanosomes are transferred to epidermal cells, resulting in pigmentation of the epidermis.]*. This unpredictable reaction to skin injury(like abrasions from scratching) combined with unprotected sun exposure should all the more encourage all acne patients except Caucasians to be extra careful in in handling their acne. In the early eruptive stage, this is due to inflammation and actual bleeding from needling or pricking; in the later stage it is due to the accumulated breakdown of by-products of hemoglobin.

Clinical features and common complaints that bring patients to doctors offices are:

1) Infection or breakouts.
2) Discoloration or pigmentation of the skin.
3) Facial scarring.
4) Depression and other psychological issues.

The next section will show some schematic pathways of how they evolve. Understanding their mechanisms have helped us design a more proactive and preventive approach in our acne complication management.

What is AcneC$_X$-PLANATION?

I t is simply defined as a description or illustration of how acne infection, pigmentation and scarring evolve or develop. These are the three common acne complications that bring patients to doctor's offices although other complaints such as anxiety, depression leading psychological body image changes resulting in suicide have also been reported. When acne or acne prone individuals are made aware or educated on the cause or the various factors that contribute to the development of these acne complications, then preventative measures can be taken or formulated to mitigate these complications from happening. Short of being redundant, allow me to illustrate these 3 common complications.

AcneC$_X$-PLANATION of Infection

Acne breakouts or infection will always happen on people with acne, acne prone or pubertal individuals because of genetics, hormonal factors and stress factors involved. Treatment goal consist of preventing such infection from NOT getting any worse into pigmentation or permanent scars which are definitely achievable in well motivated individuals oftentimes without the help of a physician or pharmacist. Hence, the importance of self learning and practicing why one should not prick, squeeze or do any invasive manipulations and other preventive principles taught in this book. For purposes of protecting one's privacy, some information have been deliberately modified in the various illustrations in this book. Below is a lady in her mid 20s with acute and chronic acne breakouts for 8 to 10 years. Treatment consisted with a family physician prescribed anti acne regimen together with weekly or by weekly office facial cleansing and toning. Also has developed the habit of using harsh wash cloth and vigorous cleansing.

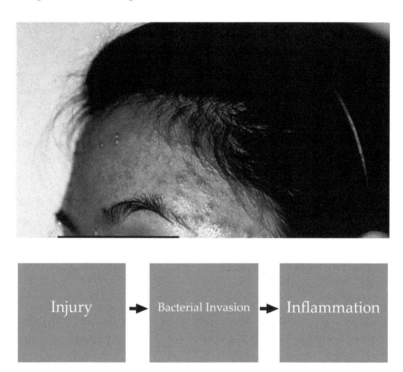

Treatment consist of quick overview of AcneCx-PLANATION of infection, gentle facial cleanser foaming gel or enzyme based detergent which loosens up dirt without vigorous rubbing or scrubbing(as in the principle of "atrophy of dis-use"), mild exfoliant, retinoid, sunscreen and discontinuance of regular office facial cleansing and toning. Emphasizing that if there is no skin injury resulting from office or self induced scratching, squeezing, pimple popping or white head or blackhead extraction, infection is remote.

A six-week result of the same patient:

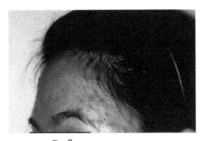

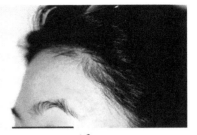

Before   *After*

AcneC_x-PLANATION of Discoloration

Acquired discoloration or pigmentation in any form or size, when it is in the face almost always command attention specially in women. The usual response or "quick fix" approach by caregivers or beauticians to this issue are skin lighteners or concealers oftentimes, both. Although we use skin lighteners as a supplement to our program, we found that after explaining and demonstrating our preventive approach to this sometimes stubborn acne complication, patients find it more predictable, natural and most cost-effective way of treatment. Our next patient is a 17 year old Latin American lady with acute and chronic zits since age 11. Her treatment consisted of harsh loofah and facial granules scrub with the misconception that such physical and mechanical cleansing will expedite the cleansing and smoothening of her facial skin. This was combined with frequent facials as well as some over the counter acne products.

Treatment consisted of quick overview of AcneCx-PLANATION of pigmentation with emphasis on identifying and doing mitigating efforts of pigmentation avoidance together with the other recommendations related to the previously discussed topic of acne infection. All these with super emphasis on the gentleness and non vigorous applications of the facial lotions and creams - with OUTMOST CARE so as not to stimulate the oil glands and avoid unnecessary trauma.

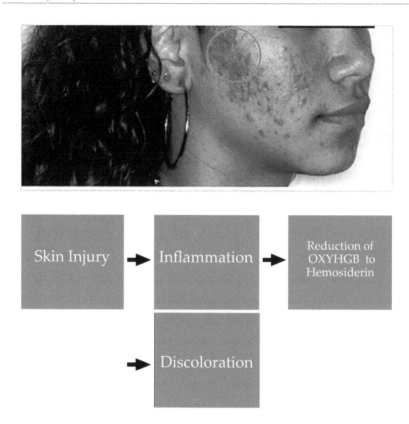

Below is a 4 week result.

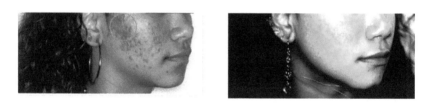

Repeated trauma causes the layered deposition *[the act of depositing]* of **hemosiderin pigment** *[hemosiderin forms after trauma or hemorrhage as it results from the break down of red blood cells. Hemosiderin causes the yellow-brown pigmentation one sees as a bruise is healing]*, thus, causing the discolorations to be more pronounced. Ordinarily, local facial vascular, lymphatic circulation absorb these reduction by-products. The **oxyhemoglobin** red color changes to brown, then to an even darker black color, if **traumatic injury is REPETITIVE**. Such injury may be as simple and innocuous as stroking, pricking, rubbing, massaging or injecting.

The **key** factor a person must remember in order to produce skin discoloration or pigmentation is its **CHRONICITY or REPETIVENESS of the trauma**. If the pricking or injury are not recurrent, the local facial vascular and lymphatic circulation should be able to handle such potential dyspigmentation by absorption of the reduction by-products. However, **if the trauma, even by scratching, becomes habitual and repetitive**, a more permanent and **deeper pigmentation ensues**. You can observe this phenomenon in individuals who have an **itchy** skin problem either from allergy/skin disease or from dryness. The patient's **skin** will just get darker and **more pigmented** as they **keep on scratching**. These **excoriations (scratches)** or abrasions of the skin **lead to** microscopic or gross **bleeding** and **subsequent pigmentations**. This phenomenon is also a common observation in areas with a high degree of contact such as the elbow and knees areas. These are common on disabled persons using their elbow, knees, or both to ambulate or get around; monks or nuns doing their religious rituals on their knees, approaching the altar. With these controllable factors in mind, acne and acne prone patients should be able to limit, if not totally avoid, the otherwise devastating effects of uncontrolled or mismanaged acne treatments. A patient who is familiar and well informed about acne and its development of complications will have a more predictable and favorable treatment outcome. When a patient avoids *chronic repetitive trauma/injury* and understands the proper use of non-prescription acne medicines and **sunscreen**, results will be very pleasing and more satisfying.

AcneC$_x$-PLANATION of Anxiety, Depression (Acne-Pression)

Anxiety or worry are our body's natural response system to an imminent event or something with an uncertain outcome which happens on acne patients particularly on those ignorant or ill informed of its nature. In general, anxiety or worry is perceived as a healthy but a temporary body response, signifying our body's immediate response to stress. It is when this anxiety and worry becomes excessive and compulsive that it becomes problematic. The recurrent and sometimes uncontrolled and unpredictable amount of breakouts in a woman's face monthly, trigger undue negative mental anxiety. This is particularly true in a looks and beauty oriented society. What may start as ordinary and simple cosmetic worry can lead to anxiety, depression and psychological overlay. If not properly addressed and managed properly this can leading to body image changes resulting in self mutilation and even suicide. But on the other hand, when early diagnosed and treated properly, this can culminate in the development of a healthy, productive and successful member of society and not a casualty. Below is a 25 year old female psychologist, esthetician, dental executive with more than 10 years of seemingly endless appearance of intermittent acne breakouts. Eruptions are even more numerous prior to her menstrual cycle and worst when expecting social events.

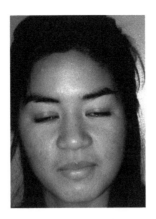

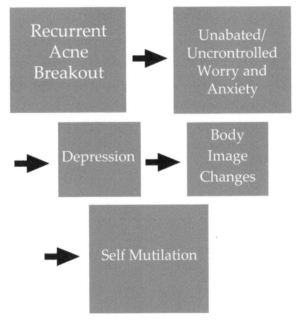

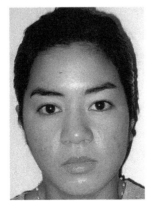

Preparatory to the next topic of keloidal scars below. Please allow me to highlight and give a word of caution on acne or acne prone patients planning on the currently vogue practice of having **multiple ear piercing,** as shown by the lady with pigmentary acne. This is in relation to keloidal development. Our ADVICE is PLEASE DON'T OR AVOID SINGLE OR MULTIPLE EAR PIERCING. This is especially true with individuals who are Black or non white. Although, fortunate not to develop keloid as EXPECTED, the multipierced ear lady is just another proof of medicine being an inexact science. Please stay on the side of caution as keloid treatment involving the ears can be both frustrating and expensive. Again, DO NOT or AVOID single or multiple ear piercing if you are a person with a skin of color. AGAIN, don't or avoid SINGLE OR MULTIPLE EAR PIERCING. If you have signs of having keloidal scar, please seek immediate medical advise as they tend to grow and destroy normal structures without being fatal. These can be safely managed and controlled when treated early and properly.

Keloidal Acne

This next patient is a 21 year old, male complaining about acne breakouts, pigmentation, scars and some "razor bumps" on his jaw areas. He has been under a physician's care with little to no success. His most important complaint was the multiplying number of razor bumps after manual shaving. These were followed by bleeding, bumpiness, pigmentation and scarring of the areas shaved. Switching him to a rotatory "pull up" shaver (electric or battery) together with instructions FOCUSING on preventing more acne complications instead of cure, the results are quite obvious in 5 to 6 weeks following the AcneCx®-Proofing Program.

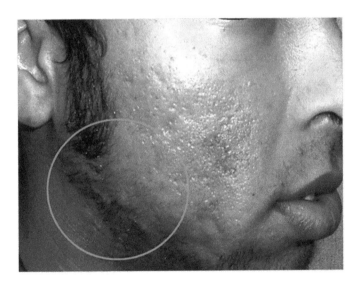

Acne/oily type of skin or acne prone individuals have been found prone to develop keloid or prominent scarring. Even **scratching** an itch from a mosquito or insect bite can develop into a **keloid**.

KELOID is an abnormal way of wound healing, which instead of healing flat to the skin surface, results in a prominent scarring that gets bumpy or elevated on the skin, as shown in the above photo. These scars are not only itchy but tend to grow when they are stimulated even with just massaging or rubbing. Hence, these bumps should be handled "gingerly". Topical or injectable cortisone might be indicated. When the area itches, it should just BE "*tapped*" NOT scratched. As a plastic surgeon, my worst **keloid** case was that of a lady who scratched an itchy insect bite on her breast bone area. She did not seek professional consultation until it started affecting one half of her breast. CAUTION to ALL patients with acne and acne prone individuals: NEVER SCRATCH, SQUEEZE OR PRICK ITCHY SITES along these **keloid** prone areas: 1. Ears, *especially earlobes*, 2) Neck, *especially jawline*, 3) Sternal or Breast bone areas, 4) Deltoid or upper arm. Needless to say, any surgery in these areas have to be done with caution and the patients properly advised accordingly.

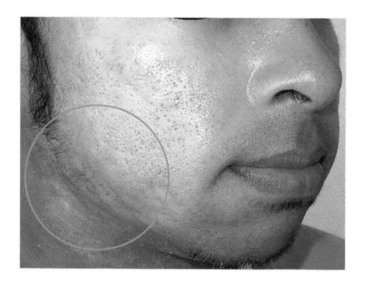

AcneC$_x$-PLANATION of Acne Scars

This next patient is a 26 year old gentleman with more than 15 years of intermittent acute and chronic acne, worst in the early years inspire of a rigorous physician supervised acne regimen. His breakouts have somewhat abated leaving him with multiple acne scars associated with scattered nodulations of white head/black head and hypertrophic sebaceous glands. After a thorough evaluation and discussion of treatment and other options, he was placed on an intensive 3 to 4 week skincare program consisting of topical creams and lotions. This was combined with meticulous compliance of mitigating efforts and rituals to prevent more pigmentation and scarring via our AcneC$^{\circledR}_{X}$-Proofing protocol followed by a medium depth TCA (trichloroacetic acid) peel. Our seven month results are shown on this patient.

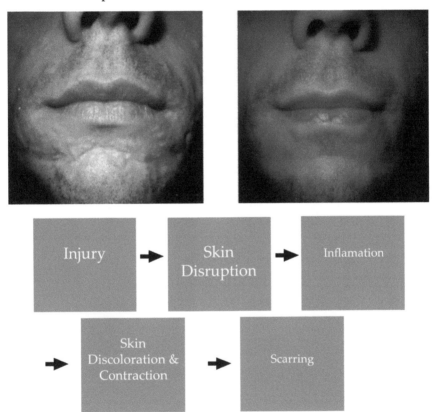

Having finished reflecting on these common complaints and their evolution or the how these complications developed into their distinct stages, did you notice a common denominator among these common complaints? INJURY or TRAUMA! This can either be physical, emotional, or both. These are mostly preventable and must be avoided at all cost. As one of our patients puts it: when it comes to my facial skin, I have learned "to pamper it like a boyfriend not like a husband!" Applying this the other way around, "treat your skin like a sweetheart or girlfriend not like a wife."

How Do We Manage Acne Scars?

From the beginning of this book, I have with special importance given detailed explanations on the merits and wisdom of using preventive measures to AVOID ACNE SCARRING AT ALL COST. Facial acne scarring, no matter how insignificant it may appear, can lead to all sorts of individual **body image problems** and social maladjustments that may result in the loss of one's life. We believe that ONE ACNE SCAR IN ANY FACE IS ONE TOO MANY!

"The best treatment for acne scars is prevention. There is no treatment that can remove acne scars completely and there is no procedure currently available that will give 100% satisfaction. Hence, when it comes to dealing with acne scars think improvement not perfection."

Can We Treat or Do Something on Currently Existing Scars?

The answer to the above question is a **"big yes"**! Our treatment goal, however, is one of **IMPROVEMENT** rather than **PERFECTION**. Once a patient has acne scars, especially, the pitted or **"ice pick type"**, these cannot be removed and are often times permanent. However these scars can now be improved significantly with high-tech or advance science methods, to the point of making these scars imperceptible. These different scientific methods, however, require a **SERIES OF TREATMENTS AND NOT JUST ONE SESSION TO GET THE MAXIMUM BENEFIT.** It is also more **EXPENSIVE** and has more "downtime". Depending on the educational training and expertise of the treating physician, the use of a single modality, or a combination of methods may be necessary to achieve a satisfactory result. These options have to be fully discussed and explained to the patient in great detail at the time of the initial consultation. Well-informed and motivated patients are easier to manage and usually obtain better satisfactory results. This is why an **empathetic NOT a sympathetic, physician** is needed with these severe types of acne. For therapy to be successful as most of these patients are psychologically traumatized, frustrated, and at the point of hopelessness, EMPATHY NOT SYMPATHY is paramount. Such concerned and **empathetic physicians** should take some time showing how scars can be improved both non surgically and surgically. State of the art and latest innovations on scar control and its improvement have to be discussed. Hopefully, these should relieve and comfort them from the feeling of hopelessness and despair, thus, avoiding some self-destructive tendencies.

Prior to discussing the type of approaches in improving their acne scars, we walk our patients thru an **overview of the acne disease high-lighting acne scar/pigmentation avoidance**. How these acne and post acne complications are developed and what makes them noticeable and prominent in plain, simple, and understandable terms. This is usually accomplished with the use of illustrations, photographs and sometimes, slide presentations.

I believe that TWO important factors that contribute to the prominence of a noticeable acne scar is either an existing 1) **UNEVENESS** or lack of uniformity of the **skin surface** in acne-damaged skin; 2) the presence or absence of **COLOR** or **pigmentation** in the proper amount; or 3) **BOTH**. This uneven skin surface on acne skin leads to unequal distribution of the sun's rays or any overhead light on the skin surface resulting in the creation of shadows on the acne-damaged skin. It is this difference of skin surface unevenness and **unequal distribution of light** that make a scar either more prominent or less noticeable.

To clarify this further, when the sun shines on a normal uninjured skin, this light is equally distributed on the undamaged skin, **EVENLY** creating **NO** shadows. Imagine the skin surface, the length of the sunbeam that will go to the bottom of the acne "hole/pit/crater" is longer, compared to the sunbeam that immediately reaches the top surface of the skin. The difference in the lengths of the two sunbeams/sun rays will lead to the creation of a shadow, thus making the scar more noticeable (See illustration below).

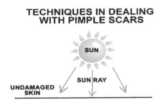

TECHNIQUES IN DEALING WITH PIMPLE SCARS

When light shines on undamaged skin, the light is equally distributed on the skin surface and creates NO shadow.

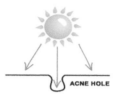

Damaged skin, like those of acne "holes/pits/craters", create a difference in the light beam lengths that touch the skin surface. The deeper part of the hole/pit/crater receives less light compared to the flat surface of the skin thus creating a darker shadow, making the acne scar more noticeable.

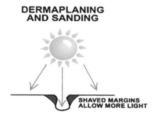

By increasing light distribution/exposure to the deeper part of the hole/pit/crater, by shaving off the margins via laser or **dermabrasion**, one can have an illusion of an improved scar because of better light distribution/exposure.

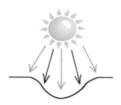

Allowing for more light into the hole/pit/crater will improve the appearance of the scar by creating less shadows.

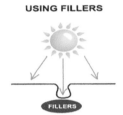

Another way of improving the light distribution on the skin surface is by the use of **fillers** using the patient's own tissue, like **fat** or dermis; heterologous tissue from animals or synthetic material can also be used. This is creatively injected at the bottom of the scar to fill up the defect.

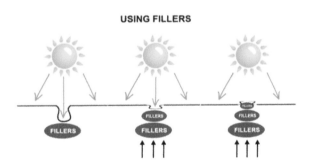

Injected **fat**/collagen pushes up the indented scars, balancing and equalizing the maldistribution of light on the top surface of the skin, giving it an improved appearance. Over filling/correction of the defect might be needed in order to counter act scar contracture and the expected long term loss of volume from absorption and degradation.

**DIRECT EXCISION
AND PRIMARY CLOSURE**

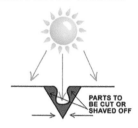

Direct excision or removal of the scar hole/pit/crater and primary closure might also be used to improve the scar (shaded area excised).

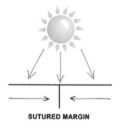

The final stage is sewing the two parts together creating an even skin surface and equalizing the light distribution. Multiple instead of a single stitch may be required to repair larger sinusoid acne scars.

SCAR EXCISION AND GRAFTING

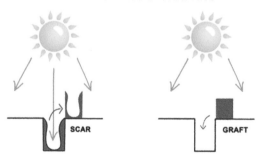

This technique is similar to the previous one. Instead of an elliptical incision, the defect or acne hole/pit/crater is cut out with a special punch instrument. This is immediately replaced and filled with an appropriate size graft from the facial area (nasolabial folds) or from behind the ears followed by **dermabrasion**.

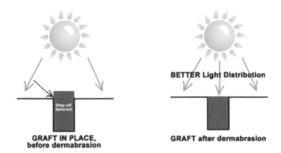

GRAFT IN PLACE,
before dermabrasion

GRAFT after dermabrasion

In a few weeks following the **grafting** procedure, **dermabrasion** or laser sanding is used to improve the texture and appearance of the graft and its step-off deformity.

To address the uneven distribution of light, one can inject collagen, fat and other alloplastic (artificial material; non living) material to elevate the bottom of the acne scar to the level of the top skin surface. Another way is to shave off, or **dermabrade (sandpaper)** or evaporate the margins of the scar with the use of laser, cautery, electrosurgery and various forms of skin acid peels, and even facelift (by stretching the skin, acne scars get shallower). All these procedures are done, with the purpose of leveling the skin surface, so that light will be equally distributed on the skin surface. These different procedures have to be performed by duly licensed and trained physicians.

How Do We Accomplish This Goal of Leveling the Scar Margins?

One of the most common approaches to improving acne scars is with the use of **FILLERS**. These are materials that are usually injected as a soft tissue equalizer to flatten out what used to be an uneven skin surface, secondary to acne scarring. This can be autogenous (material sourced from your own body) as in the case of fat, collagen, or blood components; or, heterogeneous (material sourced from a different species all together), as in the case of collagen taken from cows and pigs. Recently, soft tissue augmentations for scars have utilized **hyaluronic acid,** which are of synthetic biodegradable products of non-animal origin. The purpose of this procedure is to even-out the scar-induced irregular skin surface by initially acting as soft-tissue filler and later as stimulus for the patient's own possible collagen production. Animal derived **fillers** will require appropriate skin testing and should not be given to pregnant patients. These filler materials are mostly heterogeneous with their effect usually being temporary and will thus require a series of injection sessions to get more permanent and satisfying effect. These **fillers** will NOT IMPROVE the **"ice pick" type of acne scars**.

Although the use of autogenous **fat transplant** may seem to be the ideal soft tissue **filler** for acne scars, this procedure has not been popular for several reasons. First, the procedure requires special training and instrumentation. Second, the long term results of fat transplantation is followed by resorption (loss of substance) and degradation thus making it an unpredictable procedure. At best it may give a short term improvement of the scar, and probably the injected fat may again act as stimulus for the patient's own manufacturing of collagen.

DERMABRASION or "**sandpapering**" is another surgical procedure that uses high speed rotary instrument, with speeds of 600 to 60,000 rpm, attached to various types of heads such as wire brush or diamond fraise to even out and flatten the surface of the skin. These instruments are powered by electric or compressed nitrogen, with the latter providing faster rotation and greater torque. The patient is usually put under general or local anesthesia (with or without sedation) in a hospital or surgicenter setting. This requires specialized training and instrumentation. Even in the best of hands, a satisfactory result may require two or more sessions. Caution has to be taken in using this method of dermabrasion in dark-complexioned individuals (Blacks, Asians) because of the frequency of developing **hyper pigmentation**. This is the noticeable and obvious difference in skin tone between the treated and untreated areas. One way of minimizing this complication is to place the patient in a skin-conditioning program for 3 to 6 weeks prior to performing dermabrasion. This skin-conditioning regimen consists of a bleaching agent, **tretinoine**, cortisone and **sunblock**. The other way is to uniformly **dermabrade** the entire facial segment, with "feathering or paint-brushing" of the margins, to avoid transition or demarcation lines. **Dermabrasion** is a highly effective but "tricky" procedure that is fraught with surgical misadventures with the uneducated or even partly trained physician. Experience in the use of this technique plays a major role in the success or failure of this surgery. Hence, it has to be used with caution because it can cause more scarring if misused.

LASERBRASION is a high-tech and advanced scientific method of resurfacing the skin to improve acne scars utilizing a high-powered light to "evaporate" the outer source surface of the skin. Being computer guided, as to precision and accuracy of the depth of the resurfacing, there is less guesswork involved **as compared to dermabrasion**. This procedure requires specialization and the use of very expensive and sophisticated instruments. Patients usually require some form of anesthesia, either general or local, with or without sedation. Anybody who requires general anesthesia or local sedation will always be safer when the procedure is done in a hospital or **surgicenter** setting.

ASC Ambulatory Surgery Center. Ambulatory surgery center is a freestanding health facility that offers "in and out" type or same-day surgery. This facility is equipped with fully functional operating and recovery rooms similar to that of a hospital. **Surgicenters** are commonly used in the United States and westernized countries to help reduce the cost of health care. For dark complexioned individuals (Blacks and Asians), the same precautions should be taken as to the need of skin conditioning from 3 to 6 weeks prior to performing laser resurfacing. In spite of all the precautions, it is not unusual to still see some demarcation lines, mottled skin complexions, and **hyper pigmentations**, especially on dark-skinned individuals. These patients have to be properly advised that these reactions may take sometime to subside, usually, from 3 months to 2 years. It is imperative to fully inform the patient regarding this laser procedure, its risks and possible complications. A lot of patients unfortunately have the mistaken belief that due to the high-tech nature of laser procedures and its associated expensive professional fee compared to other cosmetic procedures, a faster almost magical type of result should be expected. That is far from the truth. A realistic evaluation and appraisal of the patient's problem, a thorough discussion of his/her treatment options and their risks needs to be done. An honest and frank discussion of professional and facility fees, will only lead to a harmonious relationship with his/her doctor as co-partners in achieving the goal of a healthy and successful outcome.

Electroridopuncture or Skin Needling with or Without Corrective or Rejuvenating Cream

In the early 1990's, a Swiss-French cosmetic dermatologist and a Canadian Plastic Surgeon observed the improvement of acne scars and other related skin problems using multiple microneedle punctures applied to the affected areas. The principle of the treatment is based upon our body's natural inflammatory and healing response to injury, in this case, the skin. The multiple punctures on the skin triggers all the stages of healing and repair which include: the release of essential tissue growth factors and enzymes as well as collagen proliferation and new blood vessels formation. This is followed by skin remodeling and scar contractility/ *(contractable or causing to grow smaller)* which results in firmer and smoother skin. Some physicians combine this method with topical creams and lotions with the intention of promoting faster healing and color blending.

Cosmetic laser machine (***Fraxel***), is based on the same principle using multiple "laser passes" on the affected acne-cratered skin. As with most laser procedures, this require a series of treatments to obtain a satisfactory result. *A Platelet Rich Plasma combined with micro needling or fractionated laser have shown promising results.*

Surgical Excision with Primary Closure, Alone or in Combination with Immediate Grafting

Sometimes, a combination of the various treatment methods might be in order, especially for the deep and **"ice pick" type of pits**. There are excised with a "punch instrument" and immediately followed by an application of an appropriate autograft of a slightly bigger size. The hair transplantation punch instruments are ideal for this type of surgery. The donor grafts can be harvested from the earlobes, behind the ears, or from the upper **nasolabial** *(of the nose)*, and **preauricular** *(of the ear)* areas of the face. My preference is that of the upper nasolabial areas, with the skin being the closest match, texture-wise, as compared to that skin behind the ear. These donor sites are easily closed with a single non-absorbable stitch of your choice. The recipient site is stabilized by **sterile strips *(steristrips)*** with no splinting necessary. A second touchup procedure of **sandpapering *(dermabrasion)*** after 3 to 6 months usually completes the treatment. **Keloidal** scars can benefit from intralesional corticosteroid injections.

Chemoexfoliation or Chemical Peels

Chemoexfoliation or Chemical Peels is the use of topical creams or liquids that have the ability to remove the different layers of skin depending on the concentration *(strength)* and frequency *(dose)* of the agent applied.

The most frequently used acids in skin peeling are the following: phenol, **trichloroacetic acid (TCA)**, and fruit acid *(alpha hydroxy and beta hydroxy acids being the most effective)*. With properly trained physicians, all these acid peels are quite effective in treating acne scars and pigmentations. Caution has to be taken in doing skin peels on dark complexioned individuals particularly with the use of the **phenol acid peel**. This has been known to cause permanent hypo pigmentation due to its destruction of the pigment mechanism of the skin. Although this can happen with the use of other acids, phenol is most notoriously associated with the permanent bleaching effect. This is why phenol should never be used on blacks. Should there be a need for an acid peel in dark skinned individuals, blacks or Asians, the use of **trichloroacetic acid (TCA)**, alpha hydroxy, glycolic acid and beta hydroxy acids will be less trouble some as to the development of pigmentary changes and scarring.

Types of Chemical Peel or Chemoexfoliation

To minimize confusion. I believe that the best and most practical description used for the type of skin peel classification is the one based on both: the frosting and skin color changes that are observed as the peeling agent passes thru the different layers and depths of the skin.

Superficial or light peel - the frost is light white and the histological depth extends to the lower epidermis[1].

Medium peel - the frost is medium-white and the histological depth is into the mid papillary dermis[2].

Deep peel - the frost is dirty or grayish white and the histological depth is to the reticular dermis[3].

The peeling agents for the superficial peels are the alpha hydroxy, glycolic acid and beta hydroxyl acids and low concentration **trichloroacetic acids**. The peeling agents are basically the same solutions but with higher concentrations of 50% to 70% for the AHA and 36% to 50% for the **TCA**. The deep peel usually utilizes phenol solution in combination with croton oil more popular known as **"Baker's Formula"**. As in the case on **dermabrasion** and laser abrasion patients, the surgeon has to precondition the skin for 3 to 6 weeks, followed by close follow up care to minimize or avoid pigmentary or scarring changes.

Herpes Simplex and Skin Resurfacing

Herpes simplex, fever blisters or cold sores are common viral infection of the skin especially occurring during periods of stress, fatigue or trauma such as in skin resurfacing procedures. They start as a reddish patch that changes into a blister or vesicle formation and then spontaneously breaks open after a day or two. This is followed by ulceration with or without pain and the resultant scar is sometimes disfiguring and deforming. This is why if there is any history of having these cold sores in the past, antiviral prophylaxis is strongly advised because of its possibility of recurrence. This **herpes simplex** which can also involve the genitals are highly contagious and direct contact with patients having open sores have to be avoided. The key to successful treatment and therefore avoiding unnecessary scarring and pain is early diagnosis and appropriate treatment. Antiviral drugs like **acyclovir** (**Zovirax**, **Famivir** and **Valrex**) orally taken and topical cream preparations have been found effective in treating both dermal and genital herpes. For prophylactic treatment to succeed it has to be given 1 to 2 days prior to the skin peel or resurfacing procedure and then continued for 10 to 14 days after the procedure. In the absence of antiviral medications, a local application of astringent such as **Domesboro** solution, a non-prescription item, can help expedite the healing thru its drying effect. This has to be mixed with water and applied as cold or hot compresses 3 or 4 times a day to relieve the pain and promote faster drying of scabs.

Meditation and Life Affirming Mental Calisthenics

There is an ongoing treatment paradigm shift in relation to an individual's physical, mental, spiritual capacity and one's over all state of health. If we want to be totally healthy especially in dealing with stubborn and recalcitrant cases (those defying standard and advanced acne treatment), physicians now offer the benefit of **meditation** combined with positive life-affirming auto suggestions and **creative visualizations**. This is in addition to the proper use of medicated creams and lotions. It has been reported that in patients who have heart disease who have been prayed over, a faster recovery has been noted on those receiving spiritual nourishment. Recent scientific studies have shown positive results in matters of health for those who practice **yoga** regularly. In our practice, we suggest **meditation with creative visualization** supplemented by repetitive verbal affirmations. Picture yourself already healed. Focus and concentrate with the "end in mind" —a healed and flawless, acne-free face. Combine this with verbal affirmations like: *"I feel **GRRRREEAATT; I FEEL TEEERRRIIIFFIIIICCCC!** I am healed."* *"My acne is continuing to improve as my body produces* *endorphins, the feel good hormones that helps me relax eliminate my blemishes."* Patients can even customized their own affirmations with words of gratitude *(to whoever you recognize as your Supreme Being or Higher Intelligence)* that you have received what you asked for. This is combined with proper medications and a skin-care regimen, at least twice a day. Do this for 5 to 20 minutes in the morning, just before rising. You might also integrate the application of an occasional clay cleansing **facial mask**. Nourish yourself with positive thoughts because the entire human race, young or old, are subject to the **"law of the farm"** *("if you plant positive thoughts: you will harvest the same in kind")*. In the same manner, negative thoughts trigger the same towards yourself. Hence, "think positively as positive results will go back to you". Because all our thoughts are within our **COMPLETE** control, why not think happy thoughts and experiences instead of negative and hopeless ones? You will feel better and happier because **one cannot be happy and have negative thoughts at the same time!**

Final Comments and Conclusion

My purpose of writing this AcneC®_X-Proofing booklet is to provide "acned" and acne prone individuals, especially the **adolescent/teenage students** *whose acne incidence is highest*. The basic information on the evolution of acne, its characteristics, diagnosis, an innovative and effective acne control starts with a well planned, achievable and realistic treatment objectives. With emphasis on methods of prevention of acne complications like scarring, pigmentations, and body image changes, results and outcomes have been more predictable and almost totally achievable. Patients have to be guided by the **TRIPLE "A" Principle** of: Awareness, Analysis and Action. Equipped with 1) a working knowledge on the mechanism of action of currently available acne **over-the-counter (OTC)** medicines, 2) practicing the philosophy of "**gentle handling and pampering of one's skin**" in **washing**, toning, the **"principle of Atrophy or Dis-use"** *"you lose it if you don't use it"*, 3) using non prescription or prescription (when needed) medications in proper dosage, and 4) allotting the approximated but essential time frame for skin repair and rejuvenation to work. All these factors contribute to achieving an invigorated, radiant and healthy skin. Therefore, one should NEVER run immediately to his/her doctor, or worst to a beauty salon, at the first sight of pimples.

Scars and pigmentations are iatrogenic *(induced unintentionally in a patient by the treatment)*. It is either **self-induced** or caused by doctor's or beautician's manipulations. If you do NOT squeeze, prick, rub, inject or even stroke your pimpled face, your chance of having permanent pigmentation and scars are remote. A few weeks of self-medication can be tried but in the absence of any significant improvement, a medical consultation should be made with an appropriate medical specialist. When the acne condition remains stubborn or unpredictable after a thorough work up, just like the ongoing COVID-19 pandemic, we should not hesitate to IMPLORE AND HARNESS the POWER of a SUPERIOR BEING, be it Allah, Buddha, The Supreme Being, The Universal Mind or The Supreme Intelligence, as in other religions. This 2020 pandemic showed the helplessness and inadequacy of human ingenuity ALONE even with the use of the most brilliant minds and instrumentations that science can offer. At times, humans have to humbly accept the need for collaboration with spiritual forces. While waiting for a specific COVID antidote and even with the now available vaccines, the strict compliance of mitigating efforts of washing, masking, and distancing can only help lower the still rising COVID morbidity and death rates. Lest our Center for Disease Control experts claim originality for their current COVID preventative guidelines, let's be reminded that the Good Lord has handed these down to His people some 3,500 years ago. Such were documented via Exodus 30: 18-21 and Leviticus 13: 45-46 to save and preserve humanity as there were no vaccines, antibiotics, or antiviral then.

This is another confirmation that PREVENTION DOES WORK! Similarly, when AcneC$^®_x$-Proofing's PREVENTION and MITIGATING efforts are properly implemented and practiced, they usually result in a more predictable, pleasing and rewarding outcome.

As a Catholic, Christian physician, I feel privileged, blessed and humbled that I can ALWAYS call on THE HEALER OF ALL HEALERS my **LORD** and my **GOD**, "Who healeth all thy diseases". HIS admonition? "AS YOU THINKETH IN YOUR

MIND AND BELIEVE IT IN YOUR HEART, SO SHALL IT BE." Teaching and encouraging patients that if you can CONCEIVE and PICTURE CLEARLY in your mind that you are HEALED and BELIEVE IT in your heart, then you will be HEALED. This powerful combination of prayerful, creative visualization and positive affirmations allow us to make the UNTHINKABLE... THINKABLE; and the IMPOSSIBLE...POSSIBLE.

Universally, more and more recent studies have shown a close reciprocal action between the body and mind, as well as the physical and spiritual elements, in matters of health and the healing process. This has led to what is called a "wholistic approach." In order to succeed, a doctor or caregiver has to address both the patient's inherent capacity to heal and the disease's removal or eradication. The latter is usually amenable to pharmaceuticals and physical therapy. The former, however, REQUIRES spiritual and mind/psychic remedies NOT always available or encouraged in our current health care delivery system. Observations clearly stated by the paragon of money and finance powered by spiritual values, Sir John Marks Templeton in his books (The Humble Approach and The Worldwide Laws of Life).

True to its etymological derivation, corrESthetiques˙ or "administered beauty" is a program we recommend you use as your safe and effective skin restoration, rejuvenation and $AcneC^®_x$-Proofing program. We invite you to try it in your own lives and pass it on to others. Properly used, corrESthetiques˙ can be a daily routine facial cleansing regimen, supplementing as an "age proofing" program in the prevention for **facial warts**, sun related skin issues, such as pigmentations, **wrinkles**, solar keratoses and sun related skin cancers. Since we are all created in God's image, each of us are all beautiful in our own unique way. Beauty is supposed to be in the eyes of the beholder. For those not endowed with inherent and genetic physical beauty, be assured that with today's technological advances in surgery, **cosmeceutical**s/ *(cosmetic and medicinal)*, instrumentations, lifestyle changes, exercise and proper nutrition, there is no doubt that beauty can now be administered the **"corrESthetiques˚ WAY."** What better time than to start NOW by embarking on a doable journey towards an acne-complications-free face culminating with your own healthy, vibrant and radiant complexion. There are NO painful injections, NO painful manipulations, NO oral medications evidence and science based **via** the corrESthetiques˚Way indirectly improved our patient's personal self-esteem through acts of helping fellow acne sufferers who, themselves, are plagued with low self-esteem and self-respect. Behavioral researchers and psychologists found that **mentoring** or any acts of helping others to achieve their personal goals, **elicit more satisfaction** as compared with self-serving efforts. Just as Christians are admonished to do "random acts of kindness", we encourage our acne patients to share $AcneC^{®}_{X}$-Proofing and "mentor" other acne sufferers, **STARTING** with a **SHIFT in their treatment objective**. And that is: from acne cure to **acne complications prevention**. Odds for success are better off, especially when the treatment program and its algorithm is complied upon. Avoidance of pricking, squeezing, injecting and other harsh, misguided facial rituals ultimately lead to NO scarring, pigmentation, infection, depression and perhaps, suicide. It is our hope and prayer that information generated from this book empowers acne and acne prone patients to adopt and develop good healthy habits and practices. When acted upon, these will result in healthy, vibrant, pigmentation and scar free faces. THINK COMPLICATIONS PREVENTION via the $AcneC^{®}_{X}$-Proofing acronym. Understanding and practicing its treatment principles can only lead to its maximum and optimum result.

Acceptance and admitting the presence of a personal medical problem, hence, a need for medical consultation/treatment. The best physician in the world will always fall short in his treatment of acne patients who do not believe or accept that they have a medical issue.

Clear understanding of the nature of the disease, which, although incurable, its complications are almost totally preventable. Hence, expectations of the proposed treatment being rendered have to be realistic. Depending on the acne character and severity, especially the presence or absence of scarring, treatment goals must match with treatment expectations. This is particularly true with acne when some caregivers aim and promise acne patients a cure when there is NONE.

Now!!! This means STARTING the program NOW. Not just learning, absorbing, discussing, but APPLYING AT ONCE the physiologic and noninvasive preventative methods of acne complications on oneself. Mandatory baseline photos taken before treatment and periodic after photos for measurable and visual progress monitoring have been essential for our numerous successes.

Exercise. 20-30 minutes 3X daily or 150 minutes per week According to Edward Laskowski, MD Professor and Co-Director of Sports and Rehabilitation of the Mayo Clinic College of Medicine, 150 minutes moderate aerobic and 75 minutes of vigorous aerobic is required for optimum results although modifications can be made according to patient's age, health status and needs. This have been proven to improve the body's over all circulation including the head area. This is due to the natural, non invasive maximum production, saturation and improved utilization of one's blood, the main fuel of one's healing energy. These incredible benefits in nearly every aspect of health, behoove everybody to develop their own exercise routine. EXECUTION and meticulous compliance of the rituals and the principles behind, mindful of what they should DO and more importantly, what they should NOT DO, (picking, pricking, squeezing, massaging, rubbing etc. of pimples) enhance the fruition of its treatment goals.

C Coach. Be a coach, collaborator or co-creator in helping similarly afflicted acne patients by sharing these basic principles and rituals regardless of what acne regimen they are on. The simple act of helping or giving alone, especially without expecting anything in return has always been followed with a great sense of satisfaction and even exhilaration on the part of the giver. This is due to the proven and time honored universal law of reciprocity (it is in giving that we receive and when you plant, you harvest).

X X - FACTOR - defined as mystical? secretive? unknown or unexplained element that makes/helps things become valuable or make goals come to fruition. My X Factor? STILL and will always be my Magnanimous, Loving and Omniscient GOD of my Catholic Christian faith. Since childhood, HE has been and   STILL IS the propelling Powerhouse going thru all the challenges and subsequent success of both my medical and non medical endeavors of helping others. Regardless of whatever religion readers are into, I can only encourage, suggest and pray that you develop a proactive and personal relationship with your SUPERIOR BEING, ALLAH, BUDDHA, YAHWEH, or Universal Intelligence in other religions. Such relationship will only enhance the resolution and fruition of your acne and other medical issues when combined with scientific mitigating efforts and armamentarium. It is therefore a balance of medical and spiritual efforts that make permanent acne complications REMOTE.

May I leave you with insights from the Book of Wisdom: If you catch a fish out of the water, it will die; when you remove a tree from the ground, it also dies. Similarly, when man disconnects from God, he dies. God is our natural environment. We were created to live in HIS presence. We must be connected with HIM because only with HIM does life exist.

Now you know the essence of our corrESthetques **AcneCx®-Proofing** success, the only complications book of its kind, emphasizing PREVENTION first BEFORE using expensive Drugs and Pharmaceuticals. THE TIME TO ACT IS NOW!! It's your MOVE!

"AN ACNE SCAR IN ANY FACE IS ONE TOO MANY!"

Try our AcneCx®-Proofing way, a proven, effective, non-invasive, painless and manipulation-free way.

Resume of Dr. J. Corres

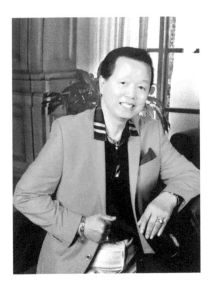

As the eldest of ten brothers and sisters of humble parentage (teacher and civil engineer), and having an average to above average mind, but a will and determination to succeed, Dr. Jesse Corres has gone through and experienced almost all sorts of odd jobs so as to get a formal education. Having a brother and a sister who were born with facial deformities, he was determined to become a plastic surgeon. Working as a shoeshine boy, selling newspapers, empanadas, or working as a jeepney conductor/barker, has taught him not only the value of money but also the dignity, honor and power of honest labor. To supplement his college expenses, he worked as a house aide cleaning, doing laundry, ironing and as in-house masseur in his adoptive family house. In school, he remembered preparing the physics and chemistry laboratories for students before and after being used, sometimes, staying late at night until all the laboratory classes were done for the day.

Now, Dr. Corres can look back with pride and humility that (together with his supportive and loving wife) he was privileged and blessed to be able to help his parents educate all his brothers and sisters. These included his two facially deformed but rehabilitated siblings (a doctor and a nurse) along with the other eight, all successful in their own chosen professions.

He underwent the rigorous training and certifications of an American Plastic, Cosmetic and Reconstructive Surgeon, with sub specialty in facial cancer surgery. He was elected President of the Philippine Association of Plastic Surgeons of America in the early 1990s as well as the President of the Philippine Medical Association of Chicago and the Midwest. He was the founding President of the International Medical Council of Illinois, a coalition of sixteen medical ethnic societies of foreign medical graduates which became a sounding board and lobbying arm on issues of discrimination against international physicians. These xenophobic issues for Foreign medical graduates (FMGs) later called International medical graduates (IMGs) were fought both in Illinois and in the halls of congress in Washington, D.C.

He later developed a skin treatment/rejuvenation program JENOR corrESthetiques® for individuals who want to look their best without laser or surgical facelift. He is the author of an acne management program for teens, tweens, and adults with adult onset acne, with emphasis on preventing acne complications. These principles and strategies were gradually adopted in the Philippines but also in the US and other parts of the world. Currently, he is a Visiting and Clinical Professor of Plastic and Reconstructive Surgery in his alma mater, Cebu Institute of Medicine, Cebu City, Philippines.

In the past thirty-five years, together with wife, Nora, he considers it a privilege and a blessing to be able to help level the playing field for those affected with facial birth defects, burns, and tumors. Yearly, free medical and surgical missions have provided these people a semblance of normal and productive lives.

In keeping with his Christian-Judaic principles of faith, Dr. Corres, together with his wife, actively participates in their own humble way by spreading God's Words and Works through various civic and religious organizations catering to the needs of the street children, the abandoned, and the homeless.

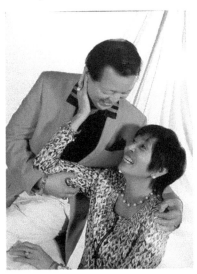

For the past decade, Dr. Corres and his wife have been blessed and privileged to work with Doctors Jim and Carm Sanchez, founders of the Hospital on Wheels in various Philippine medical missions. Their selfless and tireless efforts of serving the Philippine's poor and marginalized have inspired them to support the Hospital on Wheels mission activities, both physically and financially. We certainly encourage generous and kind hearted individuals, globally, to browse the Hospital on Wheels' humanitarian efforts. These can be done through YouTube and Facebook featuring present and past free medical mission activities, which hopefully will arouse the reader's generosity for a much needed support.

In addition, the U. S. Virginia based Montero Medical Missions is a faith based and interfaith international humanitarian organization, wherein belief in God is expressed in their hearts and reflected in their actions and deeds. Founded by Dr. Corres's fellow Cebu Institute of Medicine alumnus, Dr. Juan Montero, loving and kind hearted individuals and corporations join together to continue rehabilitate disabled U. S. war veterans locally, and the completion of the ongoing Philippine Floating Clinic. Take a look at the MonteroMedicalMissions.Org in You Tube.

Acknowledgments

Getting this book into a worthy finished product requires special thanks and acknowledgment to special and wonderful individuals.

Father Adolf Faroni, SDB, a Salesian priest from Italy, who together with Father Rocky Evangelista of Tuloy ng Don Bosco Foundation had worked for the upliftment and empowerment of the Philippines' street children and the homeless. After more than fifty years of missionary work in the Philippines, he keenly observed and noticed the very common and devastating effects of uncontrolled or mismanaged acne/pimples. It was in one of our visits to the Tuloy Foundation compound for street children that Father Faroni suggested that I write some guidelines to address, in his words, the early "uglifying effects of acne" which gave me the impetus to write this book. Part of the proceeds of this book will go towards our continuing effort to support Tuloy Foundation, which has gained the United Nation's recognition as one of the premier charity organizations in the world.

Ginny Santos — My thanks for her gracious manner, literary contribution, and the needed super meticulous attention to details, big or small, in proof reading and partial editing of our manuscript.

Milagros D. Puray, MD — An intellectual, inspiring, tireless "General Factorum" in the Filipino-American community in Chicago, Illinois. She is a U.S. triple boarded Internist, Hematologist ,and Sexologist. She exemplifies the gold standard as the "poetry in motion" type of rhyming and blending of how social, spiritual, and medical vocation and avocation should be practiced. Together with husband, Pediatrician, Dr. Cesar, the only certified sexologists couple we know, they can be dubbed as "Chicago's Urgent Care Duo" because of their ever-ready stance to help anybody in medical, physical, mental, or even spiritual distress.

Always supportive and encouraging in all our endeavors, we want to acknowledge them with great thanks and full of praise. They are not only our personal but also our family clan physicians, responsible for our entire family's health and well being. Endearingly and lovingly, we call them OUR BEST ADOPTED SISTER AND BROTHER one can ever have.

Finally, to a lovely and special couple, Leo and Narci Cruz—who for more than a decade have toiled, shared and witnessed not only the occasional disappointments but also the heart warming successes of educating the world in "RESTORING BEAUTY THROUGH SKIN HEALTH" via the corrESthetiques® AcneC®$_x$-Proofing acne and non-acne related beauty issues. Their support, loyalty, and most especially, their friendship, is most appreciated.

CPSIA information can be obtained
at www.ICGtesting.com
Printed in the USA
BVHW061514121121
621449BV00020B/699